OCN Exam Study Guide, latest with Review and Rationale

OCN Certificate Practice Questions
for the ONCC OCN test

Prof. Winifred Taylor
© 2022-2023
Printed in USA.

Disclaimer:

© Copyright 2022 by Prof. Winifred Taylor. All rights reserved.

All rights reserved. It is illegal to distribute, reproduce or transmit any part of this book by any means or forms. Every effort has been made by the author and editor to ensure correct information in this book. This book is prepared with extreme care to give the best to its readers. However, the author and editor hereby disclaim any liability to any part for any loss, or damage caused by errors or omission. Recording, photocopying or any other mechanical or electronic transmission of the book without prior permission of the publisher is not permitted, except in the case of critical reviews and certain other non-commercial uses permitted by copyright law.

Printed in the United States of America.

ONCC ®, OCN ® are registered trademarks of Oncology Nursing Certification Corporation. They hold no affiliation with this product. We are not affiliated with or endorsed by any official testing organization.

Content

Why do you need to be OCN Certified?	4
Willing To Join Our Author Panel?	5
Why is this book a right choice for you to clear the OCN Exam?	6
Magical Steps to Pass the OCN Exam with Ease:	8
OCN Exam Practice Questions	10
Answers with Detailed Rationale	77

Why do you need to be OCN Certified?

The Oncology Certified Nurse (OCN) Exam is an exclusive, volunteer certification for nurses who specialize in oncology. This national board exam provides an opportunity for nurses to validate their role as experts in the care of patients with cancer and improve the quality of patient care. Certification demonstrates that the nurse has successfully completed a rigorous examination and has the necessary knowledge to provide safe, high-quality care to patients with cancer.

As the health care landscape continues to evolve, it is becoming increasingly important for nurses to have specialty certification. Oncology Certified Nurses (OCNs) are a critical part of the cancer care team. They possess the unique knowledge and skill set necessary to provide high-quality, patient-centered care. The role of OCNs has been shown to improve patient outcomes, communication and collaboration among the care team.

Earning the OCN credential can help nurses advance their careers, be recognized by peers and employers for their expertise, and promote best practices in oncology nursing. They are often in high demand and can command high salaries. They also report high levels of job satisfaction and a strong sense of dignity and purpose in their work.

Willing To Join Our Author Panel?

Dear Registered Nurses,

We would like to invite you to join our 'Panel Of Authors'.

First of all, Thank you for your hard work and dedication to your patients. We know that the hours are long and the workload is demanding, but you do it with grace and dignity. Your compassion is evident in the way you treat your patients, and we are grateful for all that you do.

We believe that your expertise and experience as nurses will be a valuable contribution to our books. Our goal is to provide valuable content that helps nurses to step forward in their career development. This is a unique opportunity to share your expertise with other nurses and help shape the future of nursing.

The requirements for joining our panel of authors are as follows:
- A minimum experience of 8 years in nursing
- Proper certification from a renowned organization
- Good writing and teaching skills
- Enthusiasm in sharing knowledge

If you meet these requirements and are interested in joining our panel, please send us your resume along with a writing sample for our review to propublisher@zohomail.com . We would be happy to have you on board!

We are happy that our panel of authors can provide the best content because they are experienced and passionate about nursing. We would love for you to join our panel of authors and help us continue to provide quality content for nurses. You will also be able to connect with other nurses from around the world and build a network of support. Undoubtedly, this will be a great opportunity for you to make a difference in the nursing profession.

Thank You.

Why is this book the right choice for you to clear the OCN Exam?

Latest Study Guide:
If you are looking for an up-to-date study guide for the OCN Exam, then look no further than this book. This book provides everything you need to know to ace the exam with tons of practice questions to help you prepare. This book is also constantly updated to ensure that it always covers the latest information on the exam as per the outline provided by the ONCC ®.

OCN® TEST CONTENT OUTLINE (TEST BLUEPRINT)
I. Health Promotion, Screening, and Early Detection — 6%
II. Scientific Basis for Practice — 9%
III. Treatment Modalities — 16%
IV. Symptom Management — 22%
V. Psychosocial Dimensions of Care — 8%
VI. Oncologic Emergencies — 12%
VII. Survivorship — 8%
VIII. Palliative and End-of-Life Care — 11%

Experienced Set of Authors:
There are many reasons to choose this book over others, but one of the most important is that it is written by experienced authors who are OCN Certified. The authors of this book have a wealth of experience in taking and passing exams, and we have used our knowledge to create a study guide that is comprehensive and easy to follow.
With our experienced authors and comprehensive coverage, our book is the best way to prepare for this important test.

Detailed rationale for the answer:
We provide an in-depth explanation for each question, so you can understand not only the correct answer but also why it is correct. This book also gives you an ample amount of practice to help you feel confident on exam day.

Similar Question Format as that in the actual exam:
One of the most important features of this book is that the questions and answers follow the same pattern as the actual exam. This is extremely important because you need to be familiar with the format of the exam to do well on it.

Fine Tunes your thinking:
Going through the questions, answers and explanations repeatedly will sharpen your thinking and understanding ability. This will help you to understand the root of the question in the OCN Exam and make the right selection of the answer.

Clear and Concise:
This OCN Prep is written in simple language and is not overly technical. This sets this book apart from other study materials because when you are studying for the OCN Exam, you need to be able to understand the material without getting bogged down in details. This book will help you do just that. This combination of easy-to-understand language and practical testing will help you be successful on the OCN exam.

Magical Steps to Pass the OCN Exam with Ease:

1. Belief: You must believe that you can pass the OCN exam with ease. This belief will help you stay focused and motivated throughout your studies. We help build your confidence by giving you the feel of attending virtual exams in our book, making you familiar with the type of questions that will be asked in the exam, and giving you a thorough idea about all the topics as specified by ONCC ®.

2. Visualization: Visualize yourself passing the OCN exam with flying colors. This will help you stay positive and focused on your goal. Taking multiple tests and solving various questions will help improve your positivity and confidence. We try our best to improve your positivity.

3. Study: Make sure to study all the material thoroughly. Quality Learning is more important than Quantity Learning. Time yourself when you take tests and try to complete them within the stipulated time.

4. Practice: The more you practice the more is the chance of passing the exam. By doing this, you will get a feel for the types of questions that will be asked and how to best answer them. We have an abundant number of questions for you to practice.

5. Relax: On the day of the exam, make sure to relax and stay calm. This will help you think more clearly and perform at your best.

Smart Learning with Trust in Yourself will make Success knock at your door! All the Best!

OCN Exam Practice Questions

OCN Exam Practice Questions

1: While taking prochlorperazine, a patient complains of slurred speech, shuffling gait, and tremors in the emergency room. Which of the following causes the symptoms listed above?
A. Psychomotor seizure
B. Hypocalcemia
C. Heart Attack
D. Extrapyramidal reaction

2: Which of the following cancer types should Michelle, a 25-year-old woman with a BRCA1 mutation who has also had a bilateral preventative mastectomy for breast cancer, be checked for?
A. Ovarian Cancer
B. Lymphatic Cancer
C. Breast Cancer
D. Brain Cancer

3: The thalidomide-treated patient has been offered an adjunct therapeutic option for neuropathy. Based on the current evidence, the nurse's recommendation would be?
A. Fish oil
B. Glutathione
C. Acupuncture
D. Anticonvulsant medication Lamotrigine

4: Kent is a 36-year-old male with hepatocellular carcinoma and it was found that he had gastrointestinal bleeding, which could be due to -
A. GERD
B. Portal hypertension
C. Cardiac tamponade
D. Tumor lysis syndrome

5: With the help of the data about new cases and deaths of the patient with cancer in the general population, we can measure which of the following risk-
A. Risk ratio
B. Absolute risk
C. Odds ratio
D. Both A and B

6: Which option best describes the cancer survivorship plan?
A. Explaining the medications
B. Outlining the primary therapies received during initial treatments
C. Outlining the expected follow-up care after the treatment
D. Exploring with the hospice care

7: Megan is undergoing chemotherapy and her doctor was afraid of the possibility of hemorrhagic cystitis so he gave her the following drug as a preventive measure-
A. hydrocortisone
B. mesna
C. acrolein
D. cyclophosphamide correct

8: Sarah underwent allogeneic hematopoietic stem cell transplant 1 week ago. Her doctors advised her to stay in the hospital till neutrophil engraftment is steadily achieved. How many days post transplant does this take to occur?
A. 1 week
B. Immediately after transplant
C. 2- 6 weeks
D. 1 months

9: It is noticed that the previous decade has witnessed a decrease in which type of cancer incidence?
A. Colorectal
B. Bone marrow

C. Prostate
D. Oesophageal

10: Oliver was recently diagnosed with dysfunctional grief which includes all of the following signs and symptoms EXCEPT-
A. Unresolved anger
B. Anxiety disorder
C. Self destructive behaviour like alcohol abuse
D. Reliving past loss over and over again

11: Tissue damage is said to be associated with the release of the following neurotransmitters EXCEPT-
A. Acetylcholine
B. Histamine
C. Lactate
D. glutamate

12: During intraperitoneal cisplatin administration, which of the following should the patient do?
A. Medication has to be cold
B. Nothing has to be taken orally for 12 hours prior to treatment
C. Changing the position frequently while receiving medication
D. Medication has to be received under fluoroscopy

13: Ron, a landscaper, has been given a fluorouracil-based chemotherapy combination. Which of the following symptoms is the most likely?
A. Photosensitivity
B. Pulmonary toxicity
C. Gouty arthritis
D. Accumulation of fluid in lower limbs

14: Danieal recently underwent a mastectomy and informed the nurse that she is afraid to show her body to her spouse since the procedure. What should the nurse do to promote open communication in such cases?
A. Dismiss the patients worry as nothing

B. Tell her to discuss this with her spouse only
C. Educate her about the options available
D. Book an appointment for breast implants immediately

15: Gary is receiving brachytherapy and the following instructions were given to the hospital staff and his visitors which does NOT include-
A. Special protective equipment is worn by visiting healthcare workers
B. Maintain at least a minimum 6 feet distance from the patient
C. Pregnant people can also visit the patient
D. Only essential cleaning is done by housekeeping staff under nurses' supervision

16: Richard's nurse is teaching him about the patient-controlled analgesia (PCA) pump. Despite his nurse teaching him the procedure at least three times, he continued to have questions. Richard is also given a booklet by the nurse, but he doesn't read it. He claims that he cannot understand anything from the leaflet and is unsure what to do next. What will the nurse's next move be?
A. By suggesting other alternative methods
B. By starting her teaching after some rest time
C. By asking another nurse to teach him
D. By allowing the patient to practice with the kit

17: Tony is a patient with a brain tumor who has increased intracranial pressure (ICP). The most rapid imaging technique for assessment would be-
A. MRI
B. CT
C. DWI
D. X-ray

18: Dr. Megan is treating a 47-year-old patient with spinal compression of the lumbar spine and suggested a bowel and bladder management program which may include-
A. Decreased fluid intake to 1 liter per day
B. Loperamide

C. Use of an indwelling catheter
D. Lowered fiber intake

19: Leo has small cell lung cancer and is currently undergoing chemotherapy for the same. During his chemotherapy session, he complained to the doctor about weight gain, loss of appetite and nausea. His serum sodium level is 128 mEq/L and potassium is 6 mEq/L, which is indicative of -
A. tumor lysis syndrome
B. cardiac arrest
C. hand foot syndrome
D. syndrome of inappropriate antidiuretic

20: Harry, who is 70 years old, has experienced weight loss, abdominal pain, and diarrhea, also stated that his sleep is frequently disrupted by these problems. Prostate cancer was discovered in Harry's brother lately. What will the nurse be on the lookout for?
A. Neurofibromatosis
B. Spastic colon
C. Klinefelter syndrome
D. Carcinoid syndrome

21: Malignant neoplasms are characterized mainly by what type of cell growth-
A. Hypoplasia
B. anaplasia
C. Hypertrophy
D. None of the above

22: A 53-year-old patient came to the clinic with swollen lymph nodes and was diagnosed with Hodgkin's lymphoma. The definitive diagnostic test for this is-
A. CT scan
B. OPG
C. Lymph node biopsy and microscopic presence of Reed Sternberg cells

D. Palpation of lymph nodes

23: A patient's skin sloughing and tissue degradation are obvious. This is thought to happen following fluid leakage (Extravasation). Which of the following is the best option for the aforementioned causes?
A. Consultation with a plastic surgeon
B. Consultation with infectious disease surgeon
C. Application of ice pack
D. Administering amoxicillin

24: A cancer patient has erectile problems. Which sort of intervention has the most chance of helping the patient?
A. Oral phosphodiesterase type 5 inhibitors
B. Psychotherapy
C. Kegel exercise
D. Herbal dietary fibers

25: A newly diagnosed cancer patient's symptoms include restlessness, sleeplessness, diarrhea, heart palpitations, and irritability. Also frightened and worried, the patient requests nerve medicine. What is the nurse's most appropriate response?
A. Assure that the reason is due to a cancer diagnosis
B. Instructs the patient to ask for a sedative from the physician.
C. Informs the patient about the initiation of treatment
D. Ask the patient to explain his feelings further

26: Dr. Silvia's 37-year-old cancer patient has tumor lysis syndrome which presents the following metabolic patterns-
A. Increased blood potassium, uric acid, and phosphate, decreased blood calcium
B. Increased blood potassium and calcium, decreased blood uric acid and phosphate
C. Increased blood potassium and uric acid, decreased blood calcium and phosphate

D. Increased blood calcium and uric acid, decreased blood phosphate and potassium

27: Dr. Arias was treating a patient who had chondrosarcoma. Sarcomas have the following characteristic-
A. Originate in the bloodstream only
B. Originate in the mucosal lining of the GI tract only
C. Originate in bone or soft tissues like connective tissue, muscle, etc
D. Originate in the salivary glands only

28: Which of the following medications causes paresthesia and dysesthesia (strange sensations) in the hands, feet, and mouth?
A. Ifosfamide
B. Ifex
C. Oxaliplatin
D. Busulfan

29: Nurse Cally had to take care of her cancer patient who recently got a tracheostomy and that includes-
A. Check securement of the device every shift
B. Cleaning of tracheostomy site with betadine once a week
C. Suctioning for all patients
D. Checking of stoma site once a week

30: Dr. Nancy's lymphoma patient is currently undergoing radiotherapy for superior vena cava syndrome (SVCS). Nursing interventions for this patient will NOT include-
A. Checking for radiation therapy side effects like skin changes, etc
B. Relieving dyspnea by changing bed position and providing oxygen
C. Assessing patient's pain and providing intervention choices
D. Measure blood pressure in upper extremities regularly

31: Dr. Christopher was reading about the tumor suppressor gene p53 and it mentions the following-
A. Mutations in p53 are the most common genetic event related to cancer

B. It is rarely associated with cancers of the lung, breast, or colon.
C. It doesn't affect survival rates of colorectal cancer
D. Even one functional copy of this gene is enough to prevent cancer

32: Talia is a cancer survivor and according to the cancer survivor bill of rights she has all of the following rights EXCEPT-
A. Health information cannot be used for marketing or advertising purposes
B. Disclosure of your medical information to anyone other than medical staff in the hospital
C. You can request changes in your medical records
D. You can file formal complaints if your rights are violated

33: Harold is a cancer patient who was infected by the following organism, which is most likely to cause septic shock-
A. Coronavirus
B. Parasite
C. Yeast
D. Gram positive bacteria

34: Which of the following is an intrapsychic process-based coping skill?
A. Focusses only on avoidance
B. Focusses only on problems
C. Focusing on appraisal
D. Focusses on emotion

35: What is the most prevalent side effect of diethylstilbestrol treatment for a patient with prostate cancer?
A. Arthritis
B. Pneumonia
C. Bowel obstruction
D. Gynecomastia

36: A patient's prostate cancer has spread to other parts of his body. Which of the following cancer is known to spread rapidly?
A. Lung

B. Brain
C. Liver
D. Bone

37: Catherine is a 54-year-old female with advanced cancer. She complains of nausea and vomiting which may be due to-
A. Decreased intracranial pressure
B. Opioid drug use
C. Steroid use
D. Cannabis

38: Theodore is a 76-year-old male who has cancer and is currently receiving end-of-life care which includes transmucosal fentanyl which is said to -
A. Be the best short acting opioid that can be administered multiple times a day
B. Have fewer side effects than other opioids but similar efficacy
C. Provide the fastest relief to breakthrough pain according to research
D. Be best advised due to ease of administration to relieve pain

39: Karen recently got a Whipple procedure done and prior to her discharge she was prescribed the following medication -
A. Pancrelipase
B. Lactase
C. Lysine
D. Isotretinoin

40: Jennifer was recently diagnosed with skin cancer and is currently undergoing treatment for the same. Which of the following is NOT malignant skin cancer?
A. Malignant Melanoma
B. Merkel Cell Tumor
C. Dysplastic Nevi
D. BCC

41: Kelly is going to start her treatment at the hospital with Neratinib and her doctor advised her about a common side effect that may occur which is-
A. Severe diarrhea which may require medications like loperamide
B. Cardiac arrest
C. Dermatitis which will decrease eventually
D. Gastritis due to increased stomach acid production

42: Which of the following will a nurse aim to display when she has the ability to identify and appreciate differences in views, attitudes, and lifestyles?
A. Cultural competence
B. Presentation
C. Non maleficence
D. Protective buffering

43: Medical students at Harvard recently had a lecture about Cancer of the uterine cervix and the following is true related to that-
A. Often seen in young women below the age of 30 years
B. Pap smear is the definitive diagnostic tool for it
C. Confirmation of diagnosis is done by colposcopic examination and biopsy
D. HPV vaccine does not offer protection against any type of cervical cancer

44: During the intravenous injection of a chemotherapeutic medication, the patient has acute dyspnea, wheezing, hypotension, throat, and facial edema. What will the nurse's first response be?
A. To discontinue the administering of chemotherapeutic agent
B. To increase administering epinephrine
C. To decrease antihistamine
D. To stop administering oxygen

45: A 38-year-old male currently undergoing chemotherapy whose last session was 1 week ago, presented to the hospital with complaints of fever, confusion, vomiting, and breathing difficulties. The oncology nurse suspected the following medical emergency-
A. Sepsis

B. Allergy to medication
C. Cardiac arrest
D. Anemia

46: Paul was in the hospital for a week and passed away due to the most common nursing error that leads to a malpractice lawsuit, which is-
A. Medication error
B. Failure to monitor vitals
C. Error in documentation
D. Failure to call a physician for timely assistance

47: William needs frequent platelet transfusions and may develop antibodies, necessitating the use of additional products like?
A. Leukoreduced
B. Low body mass index
C. Reduced volume
D. Delayed

48: Leonard is currently using the following drug which is least likely to cause peripheral neuropathy and hearing loss-
A. Oxaliplatin
B. Arsenic trioxide
C. Vinblastine
D. Cetirizine

49: Dr. Justin is a sex counselor and he used the PLISSIT model of sexual counseling in which SS refers to-
A. Specific suggestions
B. Social stigma
C. Sex safety
D. Sickness symptoms

50: Emily is currently receiving treatment for opioid addiction which is best described as -

A. Unrestrained and compulsive use of the drug for recreational purposes or despite negative consequences
B. A need for an increased dosage to manage pain
C. Use of opioids in patients with chronic pain
D. Use of both non-opiods and opioids to manage pain

51: Oliver is grieving the loss of his mother and to support him the following is encouraged-
A. Following religious and social practices that help deal with grief
B. Ignoring the grief as with time it'll decrease on its own
C. Taking multiple medications to numb the grief
D. Stay away from any social settings till he is over his loss

52: A GBM patient is undergoing radiation treatment. After absorbing the teachings, which of the following statements would the patient make?
A. ' I shouldn't worry having a head ache. '
B. ' I shall avoid hair wash '
C. ' I can now stop taking steroids '
D. ' I might experience permanent hair loss '

53: Michele uses fentanyl patches to manage her pain from ovarian cancer. The following symptoms are reported to the nurse: Urination is difficult, and she can only pass a tiny amount of urine. The bladder is not enlarged, yet there is a pain in both flanks. She has minor hyperkalemia and is afebrile, according to recent blood tests. What is the cause of these symptoms?
    A. Side effects caused by the intake of opioids
    B. Infection in bladder
    C. Cervical cancer
    D. Obstruction in the upper urinary tract

54: During his initial recurrence, Jonas, a 62-year-old patient with CD33-positive acute myeloid leukemia, had a left ejection fraction of 40%. What is Jonas' recommended treatment?
A. Intravenous drug Rituximab

B. All trans retinoic acids
C. Gemtuzumabozogamicin
D. Cytosine arabinoside

55: Nurse Fiona was trying to diagnose the type of pain her patient was suffering from and she decided it was nociceptive pain, which has the following feature-
A. Associated with damage to neurons in the body
B. Burning may be felt along the body supplied by the nerve
C. Associated with phantom limb pain
D. Commonly arises in response to a stimulus from the musculoskeletal system

56: Daniel has breast cancer and she read that it-
A. Is the second leading cause of cancer in women
B. Has the highest mortality rate amongst all cancers
C. Has equal incidence in men and women
D. Has the lowest mortality rate in relation to cancer in women

57: Dr. Jessica recently started treatment for a 58-year-old patient who was diagnosed with breast cancer. Which of the following indicates the worst prognosis for female breast cancer?
A. Tumour 5 cm in size in right breast only
B. Absence of metastasis to other lymph nodes
C. Inflammatory breast cancer
D. Estrogen receptor positive

58: Dr. Lenny's patient who recently underwent whole-brain radiation came back after a few days complaining of headaches, nausea, and confusion. The doctor suspects that his patient may be experiencing the following-
A. bacterial infection of the brain
B. increased intracranial pressure
C. hypocalcemia
D. low blood pressure

59: Jefferson is a terminally ill 65-year-old with incurable cancer. For management of his cancer-related pain at the end of life, the following is TRUE-
A. Only opioids are used to manage pain
B. Nonopioids are used first along with adjuvants and then opioid if needed
C. Only iv drug administration is done
D. Both A and B

60: Lily is currently undergoing pelvic radiation and her doctor informed her about the various ways in which pelvic radiation or chemotherapy affects females, which include all of the following EXCEPT-
A. Early menopause
B. Vaginal tenderness
C. Fibrosis of the vagina
D. Increased fertility

61: When it comes to cancer treatment, which of the following is regarded as a modal quality?
A. It is used as a palliative measure to relieve symptoms
B. It causes less toxicity when used along with chemotherapy
C. It aims to remove only a portion of the tumor
D. It is considered the only treatment that the patient requires

62: Dr. Paul informed his patient about the various risk factors for prostate cancer and it does NOT include-
A. Race
B. Older age
C. History of prostate cancer in the family
D. diet

63: The newly diagnosed acute myeloid leukemia manifests which of the following symptoms?
A. Pruritus
B. Petechiae
C. Palpitation

D. Headache

64: Oliver has a colostomy and his nurse gave him the following instructions to take care of it which do NOT include-
A. Every 3-5 days change the appliance
B. Empty the pouch when it is ½-⅓ full for ease of emptying
C. Chances in skin appearance around stoma do not require special care
D. Clean and dry the skin around the stoma regularly

65: Which of the following causes more blisters or is a vesicant?
A. Dalcabazine
B. Melphalan
C. Topotecan
D. Dactinomycin

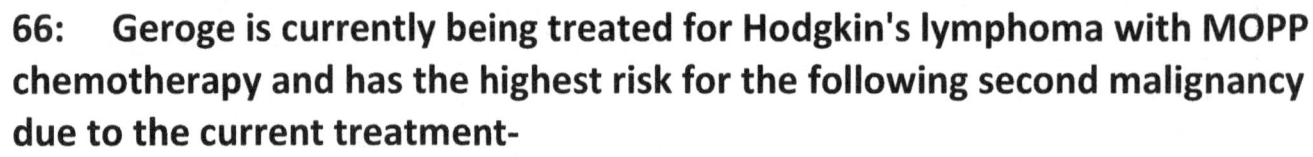

66: Geroge is currently being treated for Hodgkin's lymphoma with MOPP chemotherapy and has the highest risk for the following second malignancy due to the current treatment-
A. Lung cancer
B. Breast cancer
C. Prostate cancer
D. Skin cancer

67: Due to cognitive impairment and metastatic colon cancer, a patient is on pain medication throughout the day. The patient's behaviors are noted by the nurse: These include short bouts of hyperventilation, frequent sobbing, clenched fists, and inflexible lying. Which of the following statements best describes the nurse's suspicions?
A. Pain control is not sufficient
B. Increasing mental illness
C. Increasing antibiotics
D. Drowsiness due to pain killers

68: Nicole is a patient who requires a bone marrow transplant and the various measures that will prevent graft-vs-host diseases (GVHD) include all of the following EXCEPT-
A.   Short dose of methotrexate plus a calcineurin inhibitor
B.   Administration of cyclophosphamide and other immunosuppressant drugs
C.   Ex vivo t-cell depletion
D.   Mismatched and unrelated donors are preferred

69: During cancer education campaigns, how can the points be focused on adults with low literacy rates?
A.   By providing information in the form of a quiz
B.   Repeating the same message in a different form.
C.   Explaining the process with cartoon type illustration
D.   Explaining with the medical term for better understanding

70: Finny is receiving continuous fluorouracil infusion. His nurse regularly checks for signs and symptoms of venous irritation, what type of access is most likely to cause this?
A.   Ultrasound-guided intravenous access accomplished
B.   Port placed under X-ray guidance
C.   Repeated attempts to insert 18 gauge needle
D.   All of the above

71: Dr. Lincoln's 57-year-old patient who has a history of smoking presented with the following signs and symptoms- chronic cough, little sputum, weight loss, generalized weakness, and chest x-ray showing possible perihilar mass but clear peripheral lung fields. The doctor decided that the following procedure must be done for a definitive lung cancer diagnosis-
A.   Tissue biopsy
B.   CT scan of chest
C.   Sputum cytology
D.   Both B and C

72: Carolin had gotten a hematopoietic stem cell transplant one year ago. Infection with the following organisms is the most likely during this post-transplant time-
A. Cytomegalovirus
B. Epstein Barr virus
C. Invasive mold infection
D. Varicella zoster virus

73: A nurse noticed that her patient's implanted vascular device was flushing normally but there was no blood return. What is the first thing she must do in such cases?
A. Take an ultrasound to check the port position
B. Inject the medication even if no blood return
C. Needle repositioning and coughing of patient
D. Placing a new port

74: What is the most significant advantage of a survivorship care plan?
A. It allows the patient to have medication during chemotherapy
B. It allows the patient to make a discussion with their oncologist after the completion of treatment.
C. It provides a clear idea about the care and surveillance after treatment
D. It allows the patient to have medication during chemotherapy It will be easier to monitor the patient regarding side effects

75: Rosie, a 60-year-old obese diabetic woman, is suffering from a postmenopausal hemorrhage. Which of the following cancers is most likely to strike Rosie?
A. Cervical
B. Endometrial
C. Fallopian tube
D. Ovary

76: Which of the following should be considered in order to reduce sleep disturbances?
A. Stretching in bed and doing moderate exercise

B. Requesting the healthcare provider to stop treatment
C. Setting a comfortable bedroom temperature
D. Watching movies prior to bedtime.

77: Dr. Larry is currently planning autograft transplantation of bone marrow for his patients which has the following characteristics EXCEPT-
A. Donor and the recipient is the same person
B. Has lower rates of success than allograft transplantation
C. GVHD is not a problem
D. Healthy stem cells must be present in the patient

78: Temozolomide is a drug that is used to treat some types of brain cancers. What instructions will the nurse give to a patient starting temozolomide treatment?
A. Uncommon side effects are nausea and vomiting
B. Diarrhea is the common side effects
C. Weekly monitoring of the amount of protein in urine is necessary
D. Neutropenia occurs after 22 to 28 days of completion

79: Holly is an oncology nurse and she offers her cancer patients the following nursing interventions EXCEPT-
A. Appropriate treatment planning and execution for disease
B. Supportive and palliative care for the patient
C. Planning rehabilitation process for the patient
D. Making the patient resume work immediately after treatment

80: Kelly is a nurse whose license recently got revoked. Various reasons for revocation of license by state nursing board include all of the following EXCEPT-
A. Violation of preexisting suspension
B. Using a fake license
C. Abuse of patient
D. Trespassing

81: Harley was recently diagnosed with malignant pleural effusion and was suggested the following treatments EXCEPT-
A. Pleurodesis
B. Indwelling pleural catheters
C. Repeated thoracentesis
D. Iv morphine

82: What kind of cancer can be caused by excessive use of smokeless tobacco and alcohol?
A. Lung cancer
B. Laryngeal cancer
C. Lymphatic cancer
D. Gastric cancer

83: What is the patient's major source of information for determining the amount of pain?
A. Medical diagnosis
B. Medication for current pain
C. Self reporting
D. Monitored Vital signs

84: Jennifer is currently undergoing treatment for breast cancer and has lost 15 lbs over the last three months. How many calories should she consume to maintain her current weight?
A. 1200
B. 2000
C. 1500
D. 2400

85: Michelle, who underwent cyclophosphamide for her breast cancer five years ago, recently experienced bruises and exhaustion. Which of the following choices appears to be the suspect for these symptoms?
A. Secondary leukemia
B. Leukoencephalopathy
C. Liver failure

D.   Cardiomyopathy

86: Lisa is currently undergoing treatment for her cancer and her nurses must follow all of the below mentioned things to support Lisa's spiritual needs EXCEPT-
A.   Allowing them time and space to perform their religious practices safely during admission
B.   Refusing any sort of religious practices within hospital premises
C.   Offering to arrange a meeting with their spiritual mentor
D.   Communicate openly about spirituality and respect their choices

87: Which of the following is considered the most appropriate integrative modality for a patient with pain and a platelet count of 12000/mm3?
A.   Reiki therapy
B.   Acupuncture
C.   Massage
D.   Chemotherapy

88: A patient named Michelle has a negative BRCA mutation test result, but her sister Rosie has a positive result. When Michelle states, "I was always the difficult kid," with tears in her eyes, what emotion is she expressing?
A.   Transmitter guilt
B.   Reactive Depression
C.   Siblings rivalry
D.   Survivor Guilt

89: Sandra is a cancer survivor and her oncology nurse recognized signs of social dysfunction in her. As a process of treating this, all of the following people must be included EXCEPT-
A.   Healthcare provider
B.   Siblings
C.   Parents
D.   Neighbours

90: Harold is a cancer patient who has a thromboembolic disease which is associated with all the following EXCEPT-
A. Cancer patients have 5-7 times increased risk of thromboembolic disease
B. Cisplatin is the first drug of choice
C. Seen commonly with cancer or pancreas, uterus, and lung.
D. Risk factors include old age and female sex

91: What will be the initial step in utilizing evidence-based practices in a cancer care setting?
A. Adding all the changes in care to experience the outcome
B. Before literature research, define the patient's outcome
C. Using a medical model to explain the problems
D. Assess the patient need to define the problem

92: Jeffery underwent an ileostomy and noticed that the skin around his stoma bag appeared red and swollen after a few weeks. He went to the clinic to get it checked and the nurse first suspects the following-
A. Pouch leakage
B. Allergic skin reaction
C. Normal changes in skin and no treatment needed
D. Increased patient blood pressure

93: Chemotherapy agents act through various mechanisms. Drugs that act by inhibiting folic acid include-
A. Corticosteroid
B. Methotrexate
C. Cyclophosphamide
D. Interferon

94: Jackson came to the emergency room with complaints of severe abdominal pain. The doctor reported abnormal vital signs and on examination concluded that an emergency operation for bowel obstruction is needed. The patient was confused and mildly disoriented, unable to give consent. What should be done next in such a case?
A. Continue convincing the patient to give consent

B. Perform surgery anyways
C. Contact a representative of the patient to get consent
D. Postpone surgery

95: Nurse Tony was checking on his patient who is currently being administered biologic agent therapy. A side effect that is not normal and may require further investigations and interventions is-
A. Flu-like symptoms including chills, fever, and body ache
B. Extreme tiredness
C. Rash at the injection site
D. Sustained fever which does not improve with paracetamol consumption also

96: Charles was just diagnosed with pancreatic invasive ductal adenocarcinoma. After being diagnosed, the condition will most likely:
A. Demonstrates the spread to the liver
B. Displays the widespread fat globules
C. Remains without spreading to other body parts
D. Metastatic to Cartilage

97: Which of the following is the most significant criterion for choosing patients for a phase 2 clinical trial?
A. The patient must have an adequate performance status
B. The patient exhausted all approved treatments
C. The patient must have physiological diseases
D. The patient should not be exposed to any chemotherapy treatment before.

98: Nurse Talia was advised to follow all the following protocols while dealing with ethnic minorities and different cultures EXCEPT-
A. Body spacing acceptable to the patient's cultural beliefs must be respected and followed
B. Provide translated material and arrange for a translator if needed.
C. Be sensitive to cultural discrimination and oppression may have faced
D. Stereotyping patients to ensure better and quicker treatment

99: Danielle is a long-term cancer survivor who was administered the following drug that was most likely to cause hepatic fibrosis or cirrhosis in such cases-
A. Actinomycin
B. Bleomycin
C. Methotrexate
D. Ifosfamide

100: Nurse Carol decided that any of the following drugs EXCEPT this could be given to her cancer patient who complained of neuropathic pain-
A. Duloxetine
B. Demerol
C. Pregabalin
D. Mexiletine

101: Nurse Bethany has noticed that her cancer patient presented with new symptoms of confusion, nausea, and blurred vision. What is the diagnostic test she will suggest for the patient next?
A. MRI
B. CBC
C. Bone marrow aspiration
D. OPG

102: What is the best effective treatment for severe pain caused by postherpetic neuropathy?
A. Propoxyphene
B. Dihydromorphinone
C. Extra strength acetaminophen
D. Amitriptyline

103: Nurse Pearl was reading about ovarian cancer and the following is NOT true with respect to it-

A. Presence of BRCA1 and BRCA2 increases the risk of it
B. More common in older women of ages 60 - 64 years
C. Symptoms include abdominal bloating, abnormal fullness, increased urination, etc
D. Cancer antigen 125 in the blood is a definitive diagnostic tool for it

104:   Nora is currently taking a 5-HT3 antagonist. Her doctor advised her to be careful as the most common side effect of it is-
A. Drowsiness
B. Constipation
C. Bone marrow suppression
D. Decreased BP

105:   Harold was recently diagnosed with cancer and he came to the clinic with complaints of pain that did not decrease on taking regular naproxen and occasional acetaminophen also. Which of the following is the best next option -
A. Stopping both drugs and starting pure opioid therapy
B. Taking both drugs plus regular opioids
C. Occasional use of opioids when pain is more
D. Stopping aspirin, and taking opioids regularly

106:   Dr. Mona is advising her patients about the various measures to prevent cancer. One such primary preventive measure is-
A. Getting regular blood tests
B. Getting yearly breast examinations at the clinic
C. Avoiding tobacco products
D. Following a keto diet

107:   Melinda is a cancer patient currently undergoing chemotherapy and radiotherapy. As a side effect of her treatment process, she has alopecia which does NOT have the following feature, which is-
A. Scalp cryotherapy helps reduce hair loss due to chemotherapy
B. Hair loss affects all parts of the body
C. Poor nutrition does not affect alopecia

D. Alopecia includes trichorrhexis, fragmentation, hair shaft depigmentation, etc.

108: Sia is undergoing a bone marrow transplant and her doctors warned her about acute graft-versus- host disease and to look out for symptoms of the same. Higher incidence of this is usually related to -
A. identical twins donating to one another
B. female-to-male donation
C. young and healthy donor
D. related donor

109: Original Penny is a 54-year-old female with a history of breast cancer. She is currently undergoing chemotherapy with paclitaxel and was suggested to do the following if she got a professional manicure -
A. Acrylic nail extensions are preferred
B. Hand peels can be used
C. Use non-acetone nail polish remover
D. Soak hands in antibiotic liquid

110: Tests are commonly used to evaluate acute changes in nutritional status as well as to monitor the dietary status of patients with cachexia. Which of the following is the most frequently observed?
A. Prealbumin
B. Albumin
C. Albumin and Globulin
D. Transferrin

111: What is the principal method of cancer prevention?
A. Self-examination of the testicle
B. Guaiac fecal occult blood test
C. Usage of sunscreen
D. Systemic estrogens therapy

112: What will the nurse do if a patient complains of urticaria and itching after receiving paclitaxel?
A. Obtaining vital signs and monitoring patients
B. The infusion of the medication has to be stopped
C. Administering diphenhydramine
D. Applying ice packs to the affected region.

113: Evan is a 48-year-old male and his doctor informed him about various risk factors for colorectal cancer which do NOT include-
A. Diet high in fibers
B. Lynch syndrome
C. Family history of colorectal cancer
D. Inflammatory bowel disease

114: Ester is a 59-year-old female currently undergoing dialysis and is also getting treated with hazardous medications. What is the instruction to be given to the dialysis staff about this-
A. Stop dialysis till another treatment is complete
B. No special measures need to be taken
C. Ask the patient to stop medication till dialysis is complete
D. Use personal protective equipment

115: Sherly, the nurse explain to her patient that the quadrivalent human papillomavirus vaccine does NOT -
A. Provide protection against genital warts
B. Provide protection against HPV 6,11,16 and 18
C. Protect against 70% of cervical cancers
D. Include vaccination of all premenopausal women

116: A medical student was reading about cancer and she read the following statement related to breast cancer in whites and African Americans which is true-
A. Overall incidence is lesser in white women

B.   Aggressive and advanced-stage cancer at a young age is equal in both races
C.   Mortality rates are higher in black women
D.   Triple-negative breast cancer has a lower incidence among African American women

118: Jeffery is undergoing chemotherapy and has to receive oxaliplatin 70 mg/m2 IV. He weighs 70kgs and is 160 cm tall. What is the total drug dosage to be administered to him?
A.   123 mg
B.   245 mg
C.   213 mg
D.   160 mg

119: Richard has been diagnosed with a form of lung cancer that has progressed to an advanced stage. He has a rectum issue, watery stools, and lower abdominal pain. The nurse should?
A.   Provide a non-stimulating laxative
B.   Initiate a bulk-forming laxative and force fluids
C.   Withhold all scheduled opioids until bowel function is restored.
D.   Administer oral laxative and probiotic therapy

120: A cancer patient currently undergoing chemotherapy reported to the clinic and was diagnosed with chemotherapy induced mucositis. He was given the following instructions for the same-
A.   Opioid medications were prescribed
B.   Chemotherapy was paused till mucositis resolves
C.   Anaesthetic mouth rinses were given and no spicy food was advised
D.   Both A and B

121: Justin is a 24-year-old boy who was treated with IV asparaginase for acute lymphoblastic leukemia. 10 mins later he complained of itchy skin, eyes watering, and breathing difficulty, and also reported a history of penicillin allergy. Emergency treatment for him includes the following EXCEPT-
A. Monitoring serum asparaginase levels and vitals
B. Administer antihistamines, steroids, or other emergency drugs as needed
C. Different asparaginase formulations administered
D. Continue administration of same asparaginase formulation

122: What is the most prevalent palanosetron side effect?
A. Constipation
B. Disturbance in mental ability
C. Itchiness
D. Hiccups

123: Ras is a gene that when mutated via the following method leads to carcinogenesis-
A. Gene amplification
B. Chromosomal translocation
C. Mutation affecting only one or few nucleotides in a gene sequence
D. None of the above

124: Mary has to undergo radiation therapy for cancer and was informed about its various effects. The organ/tissue most quick to respond to radiation includes-
A. Lung
B. Brain
C. Pancreas
D. GI tract

125: Nurse Denis was treating a cancer patient and she had to assess the patient's cancer fatigue which would help in the following ways EXCEPT-

A. Cancer treatment planning/modifying
B. Disease prognosis
C. Clinical trial admission
D. Differentiation between breast and lung cancer

126: Dr. Phoebe was telling her students about upper limb lymphedema and mentioned it has the following characteristics-
A. Most commonly associated with breast cancer and those who got axillary lymph node radiation/resection.
B. Commonly associated with men above 50 years of age
C. Treatment includes rest and antibiotics
D. Related to inguinal lymph nodes

127: Veronica is an oncology nurse and the scope of her practice includes all the following EXCEPT:
A. Treatment of symptoms
B. Patient education
C. Care coordination
D. Final approval of treatment plan

128: Wyat was advised to use barrier protection to protect his sexual partner from the following medication he is currently using-
A. 5-fluorouracil
B. Hydrocortisone
C. Ketorolac
D. Benzodiazepines

129: Recently Dr. Kelly saw a patient who was diagnosed with stage I kidney cancer, MI, diabetes, and poor renal function. What is the best treatment option for such a patient?
A. Complete nephrectomy
B. Partial nephrectomy
C. Removal of entire affected kidney plus adrenal gland
D. Removal of the affected kidney and nearby lymph nodes

130: Despite having a normal platelet count, a patient experiences bleeding gums and more bruises after two weeks of treatment. What kind of intervention should the nurse make?
A. Review the patient's history for prior treatment with ionizing radiation
B. Review the patient's medical report
C. Suggest the patient have iron rich food
D. Reassure the patient that this symptom will reduce after few days

131: Dr. Sarah's cancer patient currently undergoing treatment for the same which includes both chemotherapy and radiation complain of nausea and vomiting, which can be prevented or reduced by the following methods EXCEPT-
A. Metoclopramide
B. Corticosteroids
C. Ondansetron
D. Emetine

132: A 52-year-old patient was recently diagnosed with pancreatic cancer and is undergoing radiation therapy which is the type of cancer treatment that does NOT include the following-
A. Linear accelerator is used for brachytherapy
B. Acts by causing damage to cancer cell's DNA
C. Two types are external and internal radiation
D. Radioactive iodine is commonly used to treat thyroid cancer

133: After one week of treatment, a patient is afebrile with extensive oral erythema, white patches on the palate, xerostomia, and a lumpy sensation while swallowing. Which of the following remedies can help with the above symptoms?
A. Fluconazole
B. Amoxicillin
C. Paracetamol
D. Pan endoscopy

134: Dr. Felisha advised her 50-year-old patient on various measures to reduce the risk of breast cancer which does NOT include-
A. Tamoxifen
B. No smoking
C. Avoiding postmenopausal hormones
D. Breast examinations by the doctor

135: Radiation therapy is currently being administered to Mrs. lily for her cancer treatment and its early side effects include-
A. Radiation dermatitis
B. Radiation pneumonitis
C. Loss of the menstrual cycle in women
D. Erectile dysfunction in men

136: What information will the nurse deliver to the patient after a loop electrosurgical excision procedure?
A. To Sit upright most of the time
B. To begin an exercise program to reduce weight gain
C. To expect extreme fatigue for several months
D. To avoid inserting anything into the vagina for 4 weeks

137: After examination of her patient, Dr. Jenna came to a conclusion that her patient had carcinoma in situ which means there is-
A. Cancer with metastasis to other vital organs
B. Precancerous abnormal cells without spread to other tissues
C. End stage cancer diagnosis
D. Heart failure associated with a cancer diagnosis

138: Dr. Potter's 47-year-old patient is currently undergoing chemotherapy for acute myeloid leukemia and complained of muscle twitching, reduced urine output, and nausea. The doctor on examination of his patient noticed cardiac arrhythmia and peaked narrow T-waves on the ECG, and thus suggested the following Treatment-
A. IV calcium chlorate or gluconate
B. Increased phosphate intake

C. Higher chemotherapy doses
D. Decreased calcium intake

139: Jackson is a terminal cancer patient and he recently developed signs of delirium. The cause for this could include any of the following EXCEPT-
A. Primary cerebral tumor
B. Medication side effects
C. Decrease in tumor size
D. Metabolic changes

140: Nurse Janice carefully administers corticosteroids to her patient to prevent various side effects which include all of the following except-
A. Thinning of bones
B. Decreased blood sugar levels
C. Fluid retention
D. Weight gain

141: Poppy is a nurse who noticed the following early signs of increased intracranial pressure (ICP) in her patient which include all of the following EXCEPT-
A. Headache
B. Mental confusion
C. Decreased motor function
D. Increased alertness

142: A patient is near death. Her daughter says she wants to help her mother but doesn't know what to do. What is the nurse's role in assisting the patient's daughter?
A. By telling her to have a peaceful conversation with her mother
B. By telling her not to disturb her mother
C. By saying that her presence is enough to make her mother happy
D. By showing the daughter about the simple procedures such as mouth care

143: Dr. Sophia's cancer patient was recently diagnosed with hypercalcemia also. The common cause of this in cancer patients is-
A. Excess fluid retention
B. PTH-related proteins that are osteoclastic released by tumor
C. Increased osteoblastic activity due to tumor releasing various enzymes
D. Vitamin deficiency

144: While Docetaxel was being infused, William was immediately stirred by a doubt. He inquired as to why dexamethasone was recommended. What It prevents?
A. Fluid retention
B. Anorexia nervosa
C. Sudden uncontrolled electric disturbances
D. Fatigue

145: When a patient develops grade 3 peripheral neuropathy, what will be the primary nursing intervention?
A. Recommend for increased narcotic analgesia
B. To teach about a safe home environment
C. Monitor serum electrolytes
D. Obtain an order for corticosteroids

146: Advanced directives are based on which of the following principles?
A. Truthfulness
B. Kindness
C. Autonomy
D. Justice

147: Nurse tony performed the Romberg test on his patient who had cancer, to help evaluate-
A. Body's sense of positioning
B. Hearing ability
C. Visual acuity
D. Phantom limb

148: Which of the following tumor markers is used to check for cancer?
A. Human chorionic gonadotropin
B. Carcinoembryonic antigen
C. Prostate-specific antigens
D. CA-125

149: An allogeneic stem cell transplant cures which of the following diseases?
A. Acute lymphoblastic leukemia
B. Germ cell tumors
C. Lymphoma
D. Breast Cancer

150: Harry is currently receiving cyclophosphamide iv as a part of his conditioning regimen for his bone marrow transplant. This drug has a risk of causing hemorrhagic cystitis and all of the following drugs can be used to prevent/treat this EXCEPT-
A. Sodium hyaluronate
B. Mesna
C. Alum
D. Ifosfamide

151: Nicholas is a 63-year-old patient with a history of lung cancer with metastasis to the brain. He recently developed skin ecchymosis and epistaxis and was diagnosed with DIC. His lab reports are as follows- hemoglobin 10g/dL, platelet count of 10,000/mcL, WBC count of 12,500/mm3, PTT and FDP increased, and INR. His doctor suggested the following treatment -
A. Transfusion of platelets
B. Tranexamic acid
C. antipyretic
D. IV saline

152: Nurse Izzy's cancer patient kept interrupting her during treatment and complained saying "why did I get cancer?". Which behavior it indicate
A. Anxiety
B. Distrust in the healthcare system
C. PTSD
D. Religious distrust

153: Selena is currently undergoing treatment for her cancer and is on bed rest. She complains of constipation for the last 48 hours. What would be the LEAST useful treatment option for this?
A. Bisacodyl
B. Docusate sodium
C. Enema
D. Exercise

154: Cherry is a Malignant Melanoma survivor. She finished her therapy a year ago, yet she still complains about being exhausted. The nurse predicts which of the following stimulants?
A. Darbepoetin Alfa
B. Methylphenidate
C. Lorazepam
D. Pegfilgrastim

155: Jacob is a nurse whose patient presented to the hospital with a history of dysphagia and drastic sudden weight loss of 6 kgs in one month. What is the test he should ask for next?
A. Complete blood panel
B. Endoscopy
C. Pain on percussion
D. ECG

156: Barney is a 67-year-old lung cancer patient currently undergoing chemotherapy. He presented to the clinic with complaints of bilateral leg weakness and an MRI showed metastatic disease of the lumbar spine with vertebral collapse. His doctor suggested the following treatment order-

A. Radiation therapy, steroids, surgery
B. Steroids, surgery, altering the patient position
C. Altering patient position, steroids, radiation therapy, surgery
D. Steroids, surgery, radiation therapy

157: Zara is a cancer patient with a risk of aspiration due to dysphagia and her nurse is supposed to take all of the following measures EXCEPT this as a preventive measure-
A. Avoid rushed or forced feeding
B. Increase use of sedative medication prior to meals
C. Sit the person upright or elevate the bed to 90 degrees during feeding
D. Stay upright for 30 minutes after eating

158: After a targeted therapy, Robin reports yellow, crusty papules and itching on her shoulder. What should be done?
A. Using a moisturizer containing retinoid twice a day
B. Dilute hot bath water with half-strength Dakin's solution
C. Apply aloe Vera to the affected region
D. Apply lotion with Dimethicone

159: Walter is a cancer patient admitted to the hospital. His nurse suspected he has cardiac tamponade due to the presence of the following warning signs and symptoms EXCEPT-
A. Enlargement of veins in the neck
B. Shortness of breath
C. Chest pain
D. Decreased heart rate

160: Anticancer drugs that are hazardous are said to have various features which include all of the following EXCEPT-
A. No gloves are needed while handling them
B. Requires separate and safe disposal
C. May cause cancer
D. May cause contact dermatitis

161: Mathew has chronic dyspnea. Even at the end of his life, the orthodox intervention provided no alleviation. What is the nurse's next plan of action?
A. Asks the physician to increase the dosage
B. Discussing about the Palliative sedation initiation with the team.
C. Informs the patient about the completion of all the therapies
D. Calls the anesthetist to increase the dosage of anesthesia

162: What is the definition of proto-oncogenes?
A. A gene that looks like a normal cell
B. A gene that has the ability to become a transformer gene by transforming a normal cell into the cancer cell
C. The gene that makes tumor cells back to normal Genes
D. The gene that can provoke abnormal tumor growth

163: A hospice patient nearing death be given food and water till what point?
A. As long as the patient is conscious.
B. Until the patient becomes lethargic.
C. Until the patient begins hydration and artificial feeding.
D. As long as the patient wishes to consume food and water.

164: Difficulty distinguishing between anginal pain (progressive dyspnea), facial swelling, swelling of the neck, arms, hands, and thorax due to fluid from the tissue; distended jugular, temporal, and arm veins; disturbance in vision; headache and disorientation are some of the symptoms of a patient with stage IV lung cancer (altered mental status). The following symptoms have a diagnosis:
A. Syndrome for Inappropriate secretion of Anti-Diuretic Hormone(SIADH)
B. Superior Vena Cava Syndrome (SVCS)
C. Lung embolism
D. Compression of Spinal Cord

165: Which of the following is regarded to be the main goal in treating muscle-invasive bladder cancer?

A. Preserving the bladder function
B. Preventing the development of brain
C. Preparing the body for chemotherapy
D. Reducing the surgery time

166: **Dr. Nancy has to treat her patients with various chemotherapeutic agents. The side effect including azoospermia/oligospermia and ovarian failure are LEAST likely to be seen in which of the following drugs-**
A. Procarbazine
B. ifosfamide
C. Methotrexate
D. Busulfan

167: **Robert, a colon cancer patient, had his intestine removed and a colostomy placed. On his third postoperative day, he notices an unusual finding. Which of the following statements best describes his observations?**
A. Slight stoma bleeding
B. Moist bright, pink stoma
C. A dull, grey stoma
D. Air in the ostomy appliances

168: **Dr. Tracy is an oncologist specialist and she mentioned that many dying cancer patients complain of dyspnea which may have all the following characteristics EXCEPT-**
A. Anxiety is a common cause
B. Pharmacological management is a must
C. May include primary or metastatic involvement of lung
D. Opioids are the first drug of choice

169: **Billy is a 39-year-old who was recently diagnosed with lumbar-sacral spinal cord compression. The symptoms and signs he had were-**
A. Chest pain, arm weakness, headache
B. Neck stiffness, headaches, incontinence
C. Lower back pain, loss of leg function and bladder control
D. Foot drop, headache, neck stiffness

170: Jeffery has lymphedema and is currently getting treated with the help of compression garments in his local hospital. How does the compression treatment help him?
A. Prevents accumulation of lymph in soft tissue
B. Inhibits sensory innervations to the involved tissues
C. Helps by lowering blood pressure
D. Increases blood supply to the involved tissues.

171: Luna was recently diagnosed with breast cancer but also suffers from poverty. The FALSE statement about the effect of her economic status on her diagnosis and treatment is-
A. Poverty increases cancer mortality rates.
B. Survival rates are lower in poverty
C. Cancer screening is lesser
D. Cancer prevention is more

172: Frankie has cancer and her nurse taught her friends various appropriate methods of care at home which include all of the following EXCEPT-
A. Initial management of medical emergencies
B. Administration of medication through iv cannula
C. Management of treatment side effects like nausea
D. Changing prescribed medicine and its dosage

173: How is the cancer cell different from other cells?
A. Ordinary cells generally reside in new areas
B. Cancer cells divide only when the older cells are destroyed
C. Ordinary cells don't allow contact with the other cells
D. Cancer cells migrate to the neighboring locations and tissues

174: Elon was recently diagnosed with testicular cancer and nursing duties for such patients include all of the following EXCEPT-
A. TSE must be taught to the patient
B. Possibility of infertility must be discussed

C. Testosterone replacement therapy must be discussed with the patient
D. Patient can be advised to return to normal activities immediately after treatment

175: Walter recently got an implantable venous access device placed and the following is true for it-
A. It needs to be flushed before and after every use
B. Any needle can be inserted into the port
C. Only drawing of blood can be done through it
D. Regular replacement every six months is needed

176: Dr. Oliver placed a PICC for his 47-year-old patient and it has all the following advantages except-
A. Less irritation to small veins from medication
B. Prevents multiple needle pricks injuries
C. Allows easy repeated administration of medication, nutrition, and drawing of blood
D. Needs to be replaced every two weeks

177: Nancy is a 73-year-old cancer patient who is currently in palliative care and she reported feelings of fatigue, decreased sleep, and worry. What is the medication to be given to her for this?
A. Escitalopram
B. Vitamin B complex
C. Remeron
D. Buspirone

178: Stephanie is an oncology nurse and is currently treating a 31-year-old female cancer patient who asked her about possible pregnancy during treatment. Stephanie must respond with the following-
A. Discuss the importance of delaying conception, fetal damage due to treatment, surrogacy, embryo preservation, etc.
B. Tell the patient to get cancer treatment after pregnancy and delivery
C. Inform the patient to abstain from sexual activities completely till cancer treatment is done

D. Tell the patient it is not possible to get pregnant during or after cancer treatment

179: With small cell lung cancer, Harry has seen weight gain of up to 4 pounds, headaches, and excessive thirst. What does the signs and symptoms denote?
A. (HUS) SIADH syndrome
B. Hemolytic Uremic Syndrome
C. Pericardial Tamponade
D. Tumor lysis syndrome

180: A 64-year-old patient was diagnosed with Disseminated intravascular coagulation as a complication of his cancer treatment. His laboratory reports had the following finding-
A. High WBC count
B. Increased hemoglobin count
C. Decreased prothrombin time
D. Increased fibrin degradation products

181: Nurse Caroline had to administer biological response modifiers to her patient which includes all of the following EXCEPT-
A. Colony stimulating factors
B. Infliximab
C. BRCA1
D. Monoclonal antibodies

182: Kelly is a 38-year-old cancer patient and her doctor told her that her race has the highest mortality due to cancer, which is -
A. American Indians
B. Alaskan natives
C. Whites
D. African Americans

183: When assisting a dying patient in doing a life review, what is the ideal approach?
- A. By having a comfortable conversation with the patient
- B. By making a formal conversation with the family members
- C. By asking the regular question
- D. By asking a question without any hesitation in order to acquire more knowledge

184: Dr. Kelly follows evidence-based practice which has the following basis-
- A. Personal experience
- B. Peer reviewed
- C. Scientific evidence
- D. Fastest procedure available

185: For which of the following activities should an NIOSH-approved respirator be worn?
- A. While Administering an IV chemotherapeutic agent
- B. Cleaning hazardous drug spill
- C. While handling bodily fluids Penetrating an intravenous bag
- D. While handling bodily fluids

186: Paull recently underwent chest radiation as part of her cancer treatment. Which secondary malignancy is least likely linked to radiotherapy that she need not worry about?
- A. Angiosarcoma
- B. Thyroid carcinoma
- C. Breast cancer
- D. Prostate cancer

187: Dr. Kate is going to administer arsenic infusions to her patient. Before this, what must the doctor do?
- A. Check blood potassium, calcium, and magnesium levels are normal
- B. Pap smear must be done

C. Barium swallow test must be conducted
D. All of the above

188: Which of the following is a carcinogenic medication?
A. Furan
B. Streptozotocin
C. Anthraquinone
D. Etoposide

189: Nurse Reynolds's patient has issues related to loss of personal control which is LEAST described as -
A. Increased clarity about their life choices
B. Suddenly weeping for no apparent reason
C. Increased dependency on others for daily activities
D. Shouting at the doctors for tiny issues

190: Delirium is a common symptom of a dying patient. Is there a medication that can treat this symptom?
A. Paracetamol
B. Cetirizine
C. Haloperidol
D. Aprepitant

191: NHL staging in a 37-year-old patient revealed disease in cervical lymph nodes and enlargement of the hilar lymph nodes on CT scan of the chest. No mediastinal mass is seen and the rest of the examinations are negative, this is suggestive of what stage of lymphoma?
A. Stage I
B. Stage II
C. Stage III
D. Stage IV

192: Nurse Kelly is an oncology nurse and with regard to sexual health care of her patients, the following is a MUST-

A. Let the patient being up sexual concerns first
B. No sexual health care conversations are encouraged
C. Nurses need not have any sexual health care knowledge
D. Nurses must have knowledge about sexual health care and show a willingness to ask patients about it.

193: Justine presented to the clinic with signs and symptoms of an anaphylactic reaction which is -
A. An IgE mediated allergic reaction
B. A genetic disease
C. An IgM mediated localized reaction
D. Indicative of breast cancer

194: Among the following, who is at higher risk of bone marrow depression after radiation treatment?
A. A 67-year-old patient who is being treated for basal cell carcinoma of the face
B. A 25-year-old patient receiving chemotherapy and radiation for Hodgkin lymphoma
C. A 58-year-old patient who is receiving radiation for solitary liver metastasis
D. A 46-year-old patient receiving a boost for Lumpectomy site

195: Normal cells transform to cancer cells through various stages according to the theory of carcinogenesis, which does NOT include-
A. Gene mutations
B. Tumour promoters
C. Carcinogens
D. Programmed cell death

196: Karen is a 48-year-old female who was advised to get a bone marrow biopsy done which would help the doctor determine-
A. cytogenetic analysis
B. Beri-beri

C. menopause
D. Bone calcium content correct

197: In order to take the oncology certified nurse examination, the nurse must exhibit behavioral approval for which of the oncology nursing society's practice standards?
A. The extent to which the healthcare services are provided to the individual
B. Professional performance
C. Ethical behavior
D. Performance review

198: Larry was reading a book that mentioned cancer incidence which means-
A. The number of cured cancer patients in a given population
B. The number of new cancers detected in the year
C. The number of people who have specific cancer divided by the population at risk
D. Incidence and prevalence are interchangeable Correct

199: Which of the following references can aid the nurse in determining the characteristics and safe handling measures of a potentially hazardous medicine?
A. National Comprehensive Cancer Network Clinical Practice Guidelines in Oncology
B. The Joint Commission Hospital Patient Safety Goals
C. The Private Commission Hospital Patient Safety Goals
D. NIOSH List of Antineoplastic and Other Hazardous Drugs in Healthcare Setting

200: Dr. Raynes patient has late-stage cancer and has requested that the physician's speak to only her about her diagnosis and she will share the information with her family, which is representative of the following communication style-

A. Doctor focused
B. Passive
C. Assertive
D. Filtered

201: Nurse Justine informed her cancer patient who is currently undergoing treatment that the most important factor that puts the patient at risk for sepsis is-
A. Young age
B. Urinary catheter
C. Agranulocytosis
D. Old age

202: After four days of treatment, what kind of chemotherapy-induced nausea does the patient have?
A. Refractory
B. Delayed
C. Acute
D. Prolonged

203: Anthracycline DNA binding drug doxorubicin was given intravenously to a patient with breast cancer. Soon after, the patient began to experience swelling, redness, itching, and vesicles at the IV insertion site. After quitting the drug, the nurse should do the following steps:
A. The nurse should apply some ice and administer dexrazoxane.
B. The nurse should apply some heat and administer dexrazoxane.
C. The nurse should apply some heat and administer dimethyl sulfoxide.
D. The nurse should apply some ice and administer dimethyl sulfoxide

204: Daratumumab was administered to Kelly 2 months ago and requires a blood transfusion now. What should the nurse do first?
A. Wait till Daratumumab is completely eliminated from the body
B. Nothing special needs to be done and routine procedures can be followed
C. Suggest administration of prophylactic antibiotics

D. Inform the blood transfusion center about the patient's use of this drug

205: Pearl is a 48-year-old woman who came to the clinic complaining of weakness, constipation and confusion. She has a history of hormone negative stage II breast cancer and mastectomy with radiation therapy 1 year ago and her current ECG showed prolonged PR and QRS intervals, and bradycardia. Her chest x-ray is normal and a bone scan has to be done. The patient's symptoms are indicative of -
A. Heart attack
B. Bone metastases and hypercalcemia
C. Hypercalcaemia due to renal failure
D. Vitamin D deficiency

206: Callie is a 46-year-old female recently diagnosed with gastric cancer. Which of the following staging will mean the worst prognosis for her?
A. T3N1M0
B. T3N2M1
C. T2N0M0
D. T3N0M0

207: Ivan got a gastrectomy done 4 days ago and is now being asked to undergo a swallow study which helps-
A. Assess for possible anastomotic leak
B. Hasten recovery
C. Check for residual disease
D. Assess pathway for obstructions

208: Pearl is a medical student discussing terminal sedation for dying patients, which the following is TRUE in this case-
A. Is the same as physician assisted suicide
B. Is intended to relieve refractory symptoms in dying patients
C. Does not require patient's or family's approval
D. Carried out at home

209: Malignant cells are said to have the following characteristics EXCLUDING-
A. Sustained cell division
B. Apoptosis
C. Sustained angiogenesis
D. Tissue invasion

210: Dr. Ellis was reading about multiple myeloma and the following is NOT true related to it-
A. it is more common in males
B. Symptoms include bone pain, weakness, frequent infections, weight loss, etc.
C. Blood reports show normal RBC and calcium levels
D. Stem cell transplant is a common treatment option

211: Dr. Oliver informed his patient that the following is most likely to lead to pulmonary toxicity and care must be taken-
A. Angiotensin-converting enzyme inhibitors
B. Amifostine
C. Radiation therapy
D. Iv saline

212: Dr. Joseph's patient was recently successfully treated for cancer and is looking for employment opportunities. The federal laws that protect such people include all EXCEPT-
A. The American with disabilities act (ADA)
B. The federal rehabilitation act
C. The family and medical leave act (FMLA)
D. The warn act

213: Daniel recently got a blood test done and got the following reports- white blood cell count of 500/mm3 with 32% polysegmented neutrophils and 7% bands. What is his absolute neutrophil count ?
A. 100/mm3

B. 145/mm3
C. 195/mm3
D. 350/mm3 correct

214: Patients must normally sign a consent form before beginning the chemotherapy process. He has a concern about the treatment. What is the nurse's plan now?
A. Begins to administer while explaining the treatment
B. Addresses patient's concerns before starting the treatment
C. Ensures of getting the consent form signed and beginning the treatment
D. Asks the healthcare general to explain the treatment

215: Velma recently got a CVAD placed and she was informed about the various complications associated with it. The most common complication is-
A. Nerve injury
B. Infection at site and systemic
C. Air embolism
D. phlebitis

216: Kelly is a 38-year-old cancer patient with hypercalcemia which is common with various cancer, and is most likely due to the following reason in those with advanced breast cancer or multiple myeloma-
A. Increased vitamin D levels
B. Osteolytic bone metastases
C. PTHrP suppression
D. Increased vitamin B12 levels

217: Pauline was recently diagnosed with stage 3 breast cancer and was looking into CAM therapy, which stand for-
A. Complementary and alternative medicine
B. Corrective and advanced mastectomy
C. Chemotherapy and alternative medicine
D. Chemotherapy and advanced mastectomy

218: Which of the following statements appropriately describes the usage of a spouse as a translator for a patient who does not speak English?
A. Translation by the patient's spouse is not recommended
B. Translation is allowed only when the professional is not available
C. Translation by a spouse can generally increase the patient's confidence level
D. Translation is allowed only when the spouse clears a qualification test

219: A breast cancer survivor sobs to a nurse, claiming she didn't expect to develop lymphedema. What will the nurse's reaction be to the patient?
A. By taking a recent history to identify the occurrence of lymphedema
B. By teaching the prevention methods of lymphedema recurrence
C. By allowing the patient to express her feelings
D. By assuring the quick recovery of lymphedema

220: Dr. Harry was explaining to his students about immunity and intracellular destruction of microbes. Which type of immunity is responsible for that?
A. innate immunity
B. humoral
C. cell-mediated
D. none of the above

221: Penelope was looking for a biosimilar medication to treat her current illness. What are these drugs actually?
A. An identical drug that costs less
B. A medication that is made from all-natural ingredients and has the same efficacy
C. A highly similar medication that has the same therapeutic and clinical effects.
D. A similar medication that has no proven efficacy

222: Dr. Harold wishes to have a collaborative relationship with his colleagues and the various barriers for this include all of the following EXCEPT-
A. Gender, race or class based prejudice
B. Same goal of team members
C. Lack of commitment of team members
D. Legal liability for others decisions

223: Benjamin recently underwent radical cystectomy for bladder cancer and urinary diversion. The urinary diversion most commonly associated with UTI and/or renal stones is-
A. Kock pouch neobladder
B. Ileal conduit
C. cutaneous continent diversion
D. Ureteral stent

224: What function is maintained by the cells that give rise to oligodendroglia tumors?
A. Cell body
B. Myelin sheath
C. Synovial fluid
D. Pericardial fluid

225: Sarah is a cancer patient receiving high-dose cytarabine chemotherapy. Prior to her taking the drug, the nurse asks the patient to perform various tasks which include-
A. Writing the first and last name
B. Walking for 5 mins and checking respiratory rate
C. Check blood sugar levels
D. Urine sample given to check for ketones

226: Robert, a 19-year-old patient with testicular cancer who will be treated with cisplatin and pelvic radiation, is concerned about his ability to conceive children. The nurse will make a recommendation for Robert ?
A. Preserving the sperm before initiating the treatment

B. After the completion of the treatment, sildenafil is given to the patient before engaging in sexual activity.
C. Cryopreservation after completion of cisplatin treatment
D. Sexual counseling throughout the treatment

227: Who is more prone to skin breakdown?
A. A patient with decreased serum albumin level
B. A patient with hyperpigmentation
C. Higher mobilized patient
D. A patient with decreased sensory perception

228: Dr. Veronica suspects her pregnant patient may have cancer. What is the safest and most reliable diagnostic method to use in this case?
A. CT
B. MRI
C. IOPA
D. Nuclear imaging

229: Billy is a 63-year-old diagnosed with cancer. He complained of pain and so his nurse decided to do an assessment of it which included all of the conditions EXCEPT-
A. Aggravating factors
B. Alleviating factors
C. Duration of pain
D. Patients emotions about pain

230: Jackson was recently diagnosed with prostate cancer which has the following characteristics EXCEPT-
A. Screening tests done include DRE and PSA test
B. Symptoms include trouble urinating, blood in urine, decreased force in the urine stream, etc.
C. Black people have an increased risk for it
D. Its commonly seen in those below 40 years of age

231: Nurse Lily gave her patient ondansetron which is known to act as an-
A. Anticonvulsant
B. Osteoblastic agent
C. Vitamin B complex component
D. Antiemetic

232: Letrozole is currently being given to Jenifer to treat her breast cancer and she is premenopausal. Ovarian ablation is also a suggested treatment using the following drug-
A. Goserelin
B. Firmago
C. Hydrocortisone
D. Cetrorelix

233: Which of the following is considered to react to treatment with interleukin-2?
A. Accumulation of abnormal B lymphocyte
B. Advanced testicular cancer
C. Urothelial carcinoma
D. Metastatic melanoma

234: With respect to B lymphocytes the following is true-
A. Are associated with humoral immunity
B. Mature in the thymus
C. Are associated with cellular immunity
D. Do not affect t lymphocytes functioning at all

235: The carcinogen that is NOT a sources of radiation is-
A. Chest x ray
B. Cosmic radiation
C. Radioactive gas radon
D. Asbestos

236: Caleb was informed about the risk factors and preventive measures associated with colon cancer by his doctor. One such modifiable risk factor for colon cancer is-
A. Race
B. Genetics
C. Age
D. Diet

237: Which of the following can happen if a patient's end-of-life care is neglected?
A. Sense of peace
B. Hopes to recovery
C. Adequate pain control
D. Premature death

238: William's cancer has spread widely. He claims, "I refuse to be treated. Anyway, because I'm going to die, I'd rather spend it with my family ", What will the nurse's intervention be?
A. " Completing your treatment is more important"
B. " You will definitely feel better tomorrow"
C. " Did you discuss this with your support group?"
D. " Would you like to discuss about the hospice service?"

239: For some weeks, Robin has been suffering from a persistent depression condition (dysthymic behavior). What should the nurse look for first?
A. Cognitive learning
B. Recurrence of disease
C. Depression
D. Bowel Habits

240: Various methods followed during surgical treatment of cancer to prevent further spread of cancer include all of the following EXCEPT-
A. Removal of normal tissue around the surgical margin

B. No touch isolation technique
C. Using less invasive methods like laparoscopy
D. Cutting into the center of the tumor

241: Various studies report that lifestyle changes and screening helps prevent the following percentage of cancer related deaths-
A. 20%
B. 10%
C. 50%
D. 45%

242: Caroline is currently receiving palliative care for her cancer and the following is true related to it-
A. Offered only at home
B. Done only when disease treatment is discontinued
C. Meant to provide relief from symptoms and stress of illness
D. Provided only by trained nurses

243: Alicia is a 57-year-old patient with a history of breast cancer and was recently diagnosed with malignant pericardial effusion which has all the following features EXCEPT-
A. Associated with dyspnea, cough and chest pain
B. Not associated with lung cancer or breast cancer
C. Diagnostic tools include x-ray, ECG, cytological examination of pericardial fluid after biopsy
D. Severe cases may cause cardiac tamponade

244: What causes lung cancer the most?
A. Exposure to chemical waste.
B. Exposure to direct or secondary tobacco smoke.
C. Genetic mutation
D. Exposure to ultraviolet rays from the sun.

245: Some people are in danger of receiving inadequate pain management as they near the end of their lives. Which of the following is correct?
A. Men
B. Younger adults
C. Elderly people
D. Diabetic patient

246: Despite of Robert's alertness in making decisions, Robert's son insists on making all of the decisions surrounding his father's care. What will the nurse's appropriate response be?
A. By suggesting motivation groups
B. To ask his son not to interfere in Robert's decision
C. To arrange a meeting with family members and health care members to discuss patient's wish
D. By allowing his son to make decisions

247: Every four hours, William, a prostate cancer patient, takes oxycodone orally for pain management. During a home visit, a nurse notices that the patient hasn't had a bowel movement in 3 days and is experiencing constant and dull back discomfort. What do you think these signs mean?
A. Impending spinal cord compression
B. Adverse effect of oxycodone
C. Excess abdominal fluid (Ascites)
D. Hypocalcemia

248: After getting surgery for esophageal cancer, a patient complains of nausea and diarrhea soon after eating and was suggested the following by his doctor-
A. Eating only 3 large meals a day and chewing properly
B. Having frequent sips of water throughout the day
C. Having small meals, scheduled liquids and chewing properly
D. Following a high fat and low carb diet

249: When oral contraceptive pills are used for more than 5 years, what sort of cancer can be avoided?
A. Ovarian cancer
B. Endometrial cancer
C. Lung cancer
D. Breast cancer

250: A patient refuses to take painkillers because pain is an inevitable part of life. What will the nurse say in response to this?
A. Referring pain to the chaplain
B. Requesting an evaluation from the pain service
C. Exploring the meaning of pain with the patient
D. Schedule a visit with CanSurmount volunteer

251: Opioids are commonly used to treat severe pain in cancer patients. What can be done if a patient suddenly develops itching (pruritus)?
A. Antihistamines
B. Aspirin
C. Antipyretics
D. Celexa

252: Tesha is undergoing chemotherapy with aromatase inhibitors and her doctors are being cautious of the drug's late effects which may cause-
A. infertility
B. osteoporosis
C. menstrual irregularities
D. fever

253: Stuart was recently diagnosed with Hodgkin's lymphoma. The treatment he is undergoing is known to least affect spermatogenesis, which is-
A. ABVD
B. COPP
C. BEACOPP

D. Radiotherapy

254: Nurse Katherine has a patient who has bowel obstruction and management for this patient includes all of the following EXCEPT-
A. Encouraging a high-fat diet and bed rest
B. Keeping patient in fowler's position when needed
C. Insertion of NG tube
D. Regular auscultation and palpation of the abdomen to assess changes like rigidity

255: Due to leukemia, a gay guy is near death. His parents would not accept his lifestyle or his lover, so he asked the hospice not to allow them to visit him in his room. What is the nurse's best course of action?
A. The nurse can talk with the hospice
B. The nurse informs his parents about his unwillingness to meet them
C. The nurse can ask his parents to leave a message as they are not allowed to meet him
D. The nurse can request the patient to meet his parents

256: Walter was recently diagnosed with depression which has all the following signs and symptoms EXCEPT-
A. Feeling of hopelessness
B. Feelings of guilt
C. Suicidal thoughts
D. Increased energy

257: Janice is a sexual healthcare worker and she gave the following advice to her patient who is currently undergoing HIV-related cancer treatment-
A. Antiretroviral therapy only
B. Condom used during sexual activities
C. Chemotherapy and no sexual activity
D. Unprotected sex acceptable

258: Wayne is a 47-year-old male who was recently diagnosed with insulinoma. What are the symptoms he may experience due to this?
A. Scurvy, decreased BP, increased hunger
B. Loss of appetite, mood swings, drowsiness
C. Dizziness, gastritis, increased urination
D. Mood swings, increased hunger, double vision

259: What increases the chance of developing lymphedema after a breast cancer surgery?
A. Somatic
B. Leukoreduced
C. Low body mass index
D. Axillary node dissection

260: Jessica is a patient currently undergoing treatment with a nitrogen mustard derivation which may be any of the following EXCEPT-
A. Chlorambucil
B. Melphalan
C. Mechlorethamine
D. Cisplatin

261: With respect to conjugated monoclonal antibodies, the following is true-
A. Only radioactive substances can be added to it
B. Causes destruction of cell it attaches to
C. Avastin is an example of it
D. Both radioactive or chemotherapy agents can be added to it to cause targeted cell destruction

262: An oncology nurse is treating her 46-year-old cancer patient and with an evaluation of the patients coping skills the following should be done first-
A. Ask the patient to discuss his issues with his family and friends only
B. Talk to the patient about these feelings and fears, suggest basic coping mechanisms, and evaluate the patient
C. Inform the physician to prescribe medication to the patient

D.   Send the patient to a psychologist

263: A 39-year-old patient with a history of small cell carcinoma of the lung presented to the ER with a seizure. His MRI brain was negative. His lab test showed low serum sodium of 111/mEq/L and urine osmolality abnormally elevated at 320 mOsm/L. Dr.Harold performed the following emergency treatment appropriate for this patient-
A.   Hypertonic saline via continuous infusion
B.   Hypotonic saline via continuous infusion
C.   Demeclocycline
D.   Vasopressin receptor antagonists

264: Radiation-induced diarrhea is treated with which of the following medications?
A.   Loperamide
B.   Cetirizine
C.   Glutamine
D.   Erythromycin

265: William, who has testicular cancer, was scheduled for a unilateral orchiectomy. He inquires about his reproductive actions with the nurse. What will the nurse's reaction be to William?
A.   Oligospermia
B.   No change in fertility
C.   50% reduction in fertility
D.   Infertility

266: Jessica is grieving the loss of her grandmother and the following will NOT help her in resolving her grief-
A.   Counselling
B.   Discussing her feeling with her family
C.   Following religious customs related to grieving
D.   Not talking about her grief and being normal

267: During the infusion of Doxorubicin, a patient developed a wheel and pain at the peripheral IV site. Which of the following is considered a proper intervention?
A. Administering mesnex
B. Administering dexrazoxane
C. Heat application
D. Applying hydrocortisone

268: Dr. Jane's patient is currently receiving treatment with antineoplastic drugs for her cancer. One such drug is doxorubicin which has the following characteristic-
A. It is administered in a capsule form only
B. Has no effect on cardiac health
C. Originally derived from Streptomyces peucetius
D. It acts only by forming oxygen free radicals

269: Dr. Tony was telling his students about end of life cancer patients and mentioned cachexia and anorexia for which the following is true-
A. Only one of them is seen at a time
B. They are the same thing
C. Both are reversible
D. Both are irreversible

270: An unresectable T2 N2 M1 adenocarcinoma of the colon is being treated with fluorouracil and leucovorin. What is the treatment's goal?
A. Control in cancer growth
B. Increase in cellular contact inhibition
C. Promotion of cellular transformation
D. Radio sensitivity promotion

271: Dr. Ellis is administering granulocyte colony-stimulating factor (G-CSF) to her cancer patient which is-
A. Administered orally prior to eating
B. Can be taken by females trying to conceive
C. Given as subcutaneous/iv injections 24 hours after chemotherapy

D. Used to increase platelet count of patient

272: Lymphoma meningitis has been diagnosed in a patient. The chemotherapy medicine will be which of the following?
A. Rifampicin
B. Vincristine
C. Cytarabine
D. Acyclovir

273: Dr. Bethany was telling her students about colon cancer and the following is true related to it-
A. African-Americans are at a greater risk for it than other races
B. High-fat diets are advised for colon cancer prevention
C. It doesn't affect bowel movements
D. Stage 4 does not include cancer metastasis

274: The recently diagnosed lung cancer patient complained of mild ascites, weight gain, and early satiety. Malignant ascites are a possibility. Which of the following reduces risk?
A. Pulmonary Disease
B. Diverticulitis
C. Diabetes
D. Renal disease

275: Chemotherapy is currently being undergone by Mr. Jefferson for acute leukemia and he reported back with complaints of dark urine, muscle cramps, and nausea. What is the condition he is experiencing?
A. diabetic ketoacidosis
B. tumor lysis syndrome
C. cardiac tamponade
D. cardiac arrest

276: William is on medications for pain treatment. He has been experiencing increased constipation and stool retention. When should you help him sit on a toilet or commode to start bowel evacuation?
A. About half an hour after a meal
B. Whenever the patient urges to defecate
C. Early in the morning
D. Exactly before going to sleep

277: What is the condition that requires allogeneic stem cell transplantation to treat?
A. Multiple myeloma
B. Chronic Myeloid leukemia
C. Hodgkin Lymphoma
D. Follicular thyroid cancer

278: Shelly is an oncology nurse and she was trying to understand the patient's likelihood to adhere to the treatment plan. the following will help her in the same-
A. lab reports
B. support group
C. severity of disease
D. level of health literacy

279: Kelly has advised chlorambucil for her treatment ,she did not eat in the last 2 hours. How should the medication be given in such cases?
A. Dosage must be decreased by half
B. Dosage must be doubled
C. Dosage is administered as prescribed
D. Stop medication administration till the patient eats

280: Ursula is getting treated for cancer and has gotten the following skin lesion due to her cancer treatment-
A. Mole
B. Psoriasis
C. Erythema multiforme

D. Post-inflammatory hyperpigmentation

281: Patients diagnosed with cancer may experience death mostly due to what reason?
A. Organ metastasis
B. Pulmonary edema
C. Viral infections due to lowered immunity
D. Diabetes

282: Myeloablation for stem cell transplantation includes which of the following conditions?
A. Retrograde surgical intervention
B. Growth analysis
C. Nutritional analysis
D. High dose chemotherapy

283: Dr. Victoria noticed that her patient had generalized pruritus which is commonly associated with all of the following EXCEPT-
A. Lung cancer
B. High dose chemotherapy or radiation therapy
C. Leukemia and lymphomas
D. Liver cancers

284: Nurse Tasha has to administer zoledronic acid to her patient who has hypercalcemia malignancy. Which lab values must she check prior to this?
A. Creatinine clearance
B. Troponin T
C. LDL
D. Serum iron

285: Kelly is a cancer patient and her doctor informed her that the following treatment is least likely to affect her sexuality-
A. Radical cystectomy
B. Bone marrow transplant

C. Bilateral oophorectomy
D. Mastectomy

286: According to Dr. Derek the treatment method NOT suitable for noninvasive bladder cancer is -
A. Transurethral resection of bladder tumor (TURBT)
B. BCG and TURBT
C. Intravesical chemotherapy
D. Radical cystectomy

287: Dr. Ophelia was performing a prophylactic cancer surgery for a 29-year-old woman. Prophylactic surgery can be done to prevent the following cancers EXCEPT-
A. Ovarian cancer
B. Colon cancer
C. Lung cancer
D. Breast cancer

288: Rebecca is an oncology nurse and is required to take part in various clinical trials. The current trial she is intended to be part of has determined the safety of drugs and toxicities have been excluded. What phase of a clinical trial is next?
A. I
B. II
C. III
D. IV

289: Fiona is an oncology nurse and as part of the nursing assessment of her patient who is a cancer survivor, she included all of the following except-
A. Access to screening and other follow up tests
B. Type of disease and treatment effects
C. Support system for the patient
D. Analysing success/failure rates for various treatment options

290: A clinical trial participant made an informed decision. Which of the options below best describes his well-informed decision?
A. Though there is no positive response from family, the patient believes the process
B. Physician wouldn't have suggested if it was not suitable.
C. Gained knowledge from cancer blog and came to know about its survival rate
D. The physician has explained all these to my family

291: Dr. Davids's patient has a high risk of hypercalcemia and hence was advised the following -
A. Avoid dairy products
B. Avoid thiazide diuretics
C. Avoid strenuous activity
D. Avoid multivitamins

292: George is a 61-year-old cancer patient and he has been facing lots of issues with sleep lately. The following is true related to cancer and sleep issues-
A. Very few cancer patients have sleep issues
B. Effects of tumor and treatment cause issues like GI troubles, etc which cause sleep disturbances
C. Cancer patients sleep better in hospital setups
D. Stress due to a cancer diagnosis has no effect on sleep

293: Ophelia is a cancer survivor and her doctor suggested any of the following to address her fears EXCEPT-
A. Cognitive behavioral therapy
B. Exercise
C. Peer support groups
D. Use of alcohol

294: Nurse Denise's patient underwent bilateral neck dissection and mandibulectomy. How can she promote a positive body image for such a patient?

A. Force, the patient to go to therapy for body image issues
B. Educate the patient about body image and provide encouraging words
C. Ignore such issues of the patient
D. Tell the patient's family about the same and don't provide any further help

295: _____ is most rapid imaging technique for assessing a patient with a brain tumor who has increased intracranial pressure (ICP)
A. MRI
B. X-ray
C. DWI
D. CT

296: Whichof the following mostly causes hepatic fibrosis or cirrhosis in a long-term cancer survivor?
A. Methotrexate
B. Ifosfamide
C. Actinmycin
D. Bleomycin

297: The chance of developing lymphedema after a breast cancer surgery increases due towhich of the following?
A. Somatic
B. Axillary node dissection
C. Low body mass index
D. Leukoreduced

298: Which sort of intervention has the most chance of helping the patient with erectile problems?
A. Kegel exercise
B. Psychotherapy
C. Oral phosphodiesterase type 5 inhibitors
D. Herbal dietary fibers

Answers with Detailed Rationale

Answers and Rationale:

1:
Answer: D. **Extrapyramidal reaction**
Explanation: Prochlorperazine is an antipsychotic medication that can cause extrapyramidal reactions. These reactions include symptoms such as slurred speech, shuffling gait, and tremors.

2:
Answer: A. **Ovarian Cancer**
Explanation: Cancers for which a 25-year-old woman with a BRCA1 mutation who has also had a bilateral preventative mastectomy for breast cancer should be checked for are ovarian cancer, pancreatic cancer, and uterine cancer.

3:
Answer: C. **Acupuncture**
Explanation: There is some evidence that suggests acupuncture may be beneficial for neuropathy. The nurse's recommendation would be to try acupuncture as an adjunct therapeutic option.

4:
Answer: B. **Portal hypertension**
Explanation: Portal hypertension is the increase of pressure in the portal vein. In patients with hepatocellular carcinoma, tumor infiltration may lead to its aggravation which in turn may result in the development of collateral circulation and esophagogastric varices. These varices are fragile and easily break leading to bleeding in the GI tract. This gastrointestinal bleeding results in black stools or vomiting of blood also. Treatment of the bleeding includes iv propofol, endoscopic injection sclerotherapy, variceal ligation, etc. along with tumor treatment.

5:
Answer: B. **Absolute risk**

Explanation: In scientific terms, absolute risk refers to the number of people experiencing a specific event concerning the population that is at risk for the vent. Hence measuring the occurrence of cancer in a population through old and new cases and dividing it by the total population at risk will help determine the absolute risk of cancer in that specific population.

6:
Answer: C.   **Outlining the expected follow-up care after the treatment**
Explanation: A cancer survivorship plan is made up of the expected follow-up care after the treatment for cancer is completed. This includes information about follow-up exams, tests, and scans that will be done to make sure that the patient is cancer-free. It may also include information about the long-term side effects of cancer treatment and how to manage them.

7:
Answer: B.   **Mesna**
Explanation: Mesna is an FDA approved drug used for the prevention of hemorrhagic cystitis caused due to ifosfamide and cyclophosphamide. Mesna is a detoxifying agent which is inactivated in the bloodstream and reactivated once filtered through the kidney and reaching the bladder. Mesna detoxifies acrolein which is a urotoxic breakdown product of ifosfamide and cyclophosphamide that accumulates in the bladder and prevents hemorrhagic cystitis and bleeding due to bladder irritation.

8:
Answer: C.   **2-6 weeks**
Explanation: Neutrophil engraftment is when transplanted stem cells enter the recipient's blood and there is formation of new blood cells. Usually it takes about 2 - 6 weeks from the transplant day for your neutrophils to begin recovering. The low neutrophil count up till then means increased risk of infection and hence patients must be careful in this aspect. Patients may be hospitalised for a few weeks to ensure proper post treatment care and decreased infection risk until neutrophil count is in the normal range.

9:

Answer: C.   Prostate

Explanation: Prostate cancer is the second most frequent cancer in men after lung cancer. There is a variance in the incidence rates of prostate cancer across various regions. In countries like Australia and the US it increased during the 1980s and 1990s, however there has been a decrease since then in the last decade, which is the most compared to other cancer types. Rapid dissemination of PSA testing is said to be the reason for the decreases in the prostate cancer incidence rates. PSA screening is also said to help prevent the risk of death due to prostate cancer in older men, as the incidence of prostate cancer increases with age. However it is predicted that there will be a worldwide increase in portaste cancer incidence.

10:
Answer: B.   Anxiety disorder

Explanation: Grief is a normal emotional response to loss in a person's life. Normally it is said to include the following five stages- denial, anger, bargaining, depression and acceptance. Normal grieving includes feelings of sadness, guilt, change in sleeping and eating patterns, missing what is lost, feelings of sadness and emptiness, decreased energy, etc. There is no specific timeline for how long this process lasts but overtime the person moves ahead in life and accepts the situation. However it is said if the person doesn't even after 6-12 months move on and shows signs of grieving which include unresolved anger, extreme guilt, reliving past loss, self destructive behaviour like alcohol abuse, somatic changes like headaches, pains, etc, then it is possible that the person has dysfunctional grief and it requires intervention in the form of counselling, medications, group therapy, etc. Anxiety disorder must be differentiated with anxious feelings during grief process as anxiety disorder is a mental illness where the patient experiences constant and overwhelming anxiety in various situations that are otherwise normal.

11:
Answer: C.   Lactate

Explanation: Nociceptive pain is felt when noxious stimuli like tissue injury and extreme temperatures activate nociceptors and their associated pathways. Various chemical substances are involved in the process and tissue damage leads to the release of neurotransmitters like substance P, glutamate, histamine, Acetylcholine, etc. Various neurotransmitters thus generate action potentials by stimulating the nerve fibers. The frequency of the action potential will determine the stimulus intensity. The nociceptive pathway includes first, second and third order neurons.

12:
Answer: C.   Changing the position frequently while receiving medication

Explanation: The patient should change position frequently while receiving medication in order to help distribute the drug evenly throughout the peritoneal cavity. This will help to minimize the potential for adverse effects and maximize the drug's therapeutic effect.

13:
Answer: A .   Photosensitivity

Explanation: Ron is likely experiencing photosensitivity, which is a common side effect of fluorouracil-based chemotherapy combinations. Symptoms of photosensitivity can include skin irritation, rashes, and sensitivity to sunlight. It is important for Ron to take precautions to protect his skin from the sun's rays and to monitor any changes in his skin condition.

14:
Answer: C.   Educate her about the options available

Explanation: It is common that patients who undergo mastectomy have body image issues due the change in their appearance. This also affects their sexual relations among other things. In such cases, it's important that the healthcare workers treating the patient like nurses remind the patient that this is a normal concern and offer her various solutions to the problem including therapy, prosthesis, etc. this ensures that the patient feels heard and comfortable enough to further discuss the issue and take a suitable action of their choice.

15:
Answer: C.   Pregnant people can also visit the patient

Explanation: Brachytherapy involves the placement of radiation sources into the patient body which results in the patient giving off radiation. The amount of radiation given off by the patient depends on the dose of radiation administered. Hence those who interact with such patients must take various precautions including the use of special protective wear when interacting with patients, interactions must be short (maximum 2 hours per day) and from a distance (minimum 6 feet away) from the patient. Pregnant visitors and those below 1 year of age are strictly not allowed. Only essential cleaning is done by the housekeeping staff of the hospital under supervision and disposal of any body fluids of the patient and laundry must be done carefully following special guidelines.

16:
Answer: D.   By allowing the patient to practice with the kit

Explanation: PCA pumps allow patients to self-administer pain medication via a handheld device. For the patient to be able to use the pump, they must first be taught how to use it correctly by a nurse. Richard's nurse has already taught him how to use the PCA pump, but he continues to have questions. The nurse will most likely give Richard a kit so that he can practice using the pump himself. This will help him to learn how to use the pump correctly and understand what to do next if he has any questions.

17:
Answer: B.   CT

Explanation: Increased intracranial pressure is a neurological emergency in cancer patients. There are many reasons for increased ICP in cancer patients like brain tumors exerting pressure on the skull, tumor causing vasogenic edema, robust inflammatory reaction 3-6 months after radiotherapy, etc. There are various imaging techniques to assess the brain tumor like CT, MRI, DSA and various other advances like CT angiography, diffusion weighted imaging (DWI), functional MRI, etc. CT is considered the most rapid imaging technique which shows internal body structures like tissues, organs and skeletal structures. It is faster and cheaper compared to MRI but MRI helps in more detailed imaging.

18:
Answer: C.   Use of an indwelling catheter
Explanation: Spinal cord compression syndrome involving the lumbar spine leads to loss of neurogenic control of Bowel and bladder movements. Symptoms depending on the level of compression include constipation, incontinence, fecal retention, inability to feel bowel fullness, etc. Management included pharmacological and nonpharmacological approaches. Non-pharmacological treatment includes diet modification with increased fiber consumption to promote bowel emptying, 2-3 liters of water per day, eating acidic food to prevent UTI and limited caffeine, abdominal massage, transcutaneous electrical stimulation, Valsalva technique, etc. Pharmacological management includes the use of laxatives and suppositories like bisacodyl, cisapride, neostigmine, enema, etc. Use of different types of catheters is also advised like indwelling catheters, etc.

19:
Answer: D.   Syndrome of inappropriate antidiuretic hormone

Explanation: The tumor most commonly associated with Syndrome of inappropriate antidiuretic hormone (SIADH) is small cell lung cancer (SCLC), which leads to hyponatremia and may be due to an increase in paraneoplastic ADH secretion indicating ineffective treatment or indicative of effective treatment of cancer (with radiotherapy, chemotherapy and/or surgical removal) causing ADH to release from malignant cells during tumor lysis, due to certain drugs being used. Thus a careful diagnosis of the cause and treatment of the same must be done. Nonspecific symptoms like nausea, vomiting, decreased oral intake, fatigue, weight gain, etc.

20:
Answer: D.   Carcinoid syndrome
Explanation: The nurse will be on the lookout for carcinoid syndrome in Harry. Carcinoid syndrome is a condition that is associated with carcinoid tumors. These tumors secrete hormones that can cause symptoms like weight loss, abdominal pain, and diarrhea. The symptoms of carcinoid syndrome can also include changes in sleep habits and anxiety or depression.

21:
Answer: B.   Anaplasia
Explanation: Various types of abnormal cell growths include:
- Hyperplasia is an abnormal increase in cell number
- Metaplasia is where one mature cell type is replaced by another mature cell type
- Dysplasia is where a mature cell is replaced by a less mature cell type
- hypertrophy - there is an increase in the cell size
- hypoplasia where there is a lack of cells
- anaplasia - where poor cell differentiation i.e loss of cellular and functional differentiation occurs.

Cells may undergo these types of changes due to various reasons. Malignant tumors are characterized by the presence of anaplastic cells. Hyperplasia and dysplasia seen in cells may result in their transformation into cancer cells but not definitely.

22:

Answer: C. Lymph node biopsy and microscopic presence of Reed Sternberg cells

Explanation: Hodgkin's lymphoma is a cancer of the lymphatic system affecting those between the ages of 20-40 years and those above 50 years. Symptoms include painless enlargement of lymph nodes, fever, night sweats, weight loss, and more. Half of the cases are associated with EBV. A definitive diagnosis of Hodgkin's lymphoma involves lymph node biopsy and microscopic examination of the tissue to detect the presence of Reed Sternberg cells which are multinucleated cells. PET scans and blood tests are also done to help aid in treatment planning.

23:

Answer: A. Consultation with a plastic surgeon

Explanation: If a patient's skin sloughing and tissue degradation are obvious, the best option would be to consult with a plastic surgeon. This is likely due to fluid leakage (extravasation), which can often occur when medication is administered intravenously. If not treated properly, the patient may experience permanent damage to the tissue.

24:

Answer: A. Oral phosphodiesterase type 5 inhibitors

Explanation: Erectile dysfunction is common in cancer patients, as chemotherapy and radiation therapy can damage the nerves and blood vessels necessary for an erection. Oral phosphodiesterase type 5 inhibitors, such as sildenafil (Viagra), tadalafil (Cialis), and vardenafil (Levitra), are the most effective treatment for erectile dysfunction and have the best chance of helping the patient. These medications work by blocking the enzyme that breaks down cGMP, the molecule responsible for smooth muscle relaxation and erection.

25:

Answer: D. Ask the patient to explain his feelings further

Explanation: When a patient newly diagnosed with cancer exhibits symptoms such as restlessness, sleeplessness, diarrhea, heart palpitations, and irritability, the nurse needs to ask the patient to explain his feelings further. This will help the nurse better understand the patient's condition and determine the most appropriate course of action. In this case, it seems that the patient may be feeling scared and worried, which can be common among those who receive news of a cancer diagnosis. The nurse's response in this situation should be to provide emotional support to the patient and reassure him that he is not alone.

26:
Answer: A. Increased blood potassium, uric acid, and phosphate, decreased blood calcium

Explanation: Tumor lysis syndrome is a complication of cancer treatment where a large number of tumor cells are killed together and this causes the release of their contents into the bloodstream and leads to metabolic abnormalities. It is commonly seen in the treatment of lymphoma and leukemia. It is characterized by high blood potassium (hyperkalemia), high blood uric acid (hyperuricemia), high blood phosphate (hyperphosphatemia), low blood calcium (hypocalcemia), and higher than normal levels of blood urea nitrogen and other nitrogen-containing compounds. All this can lead to symptoms like nausea and vomiting, tetany, lactic acidosis, etc, and other serious effects like acute kidney failure, acute uric acid nephropathy, seizures, etc, and also death.

27:
Answer: C. Originate in bone or soft tissues like connective tissue, muscle, etc

Explanation: Sarcomas are a general term used for cancers that originate in the bone and soft tissues of the body (connective tissue, muscle, fat, blood vessels, etc). Signs and symptoms of sarcomas depend on the site affected and present as bone pain, lo felt through the skin, breaking of bone, abdominal pain, etc. Risk factors include genetics, exposure to chemicals and viruses, radiation therapy, etc. Kaposi sarcoma is commonly linked to HPV- Sarcomas. These are primary connective tissue tumors as they originate in the connective tissue.

28:
Answer: C.   Oxaliplatin
Explanation: Oxaliplatin is a chemotherapy medication that can cause paresthesia and dysesthesia in the hands, feet, and mouth. Paresthesia is a sensation of pins and needles, while dysesthesia is a sensation of burning, tingling, or prickling. These sensations can be quite uncomfortable and can interfere with daily activities.

29:
Answer: A.   Checking securement of the device every shift
Explanation: Care after tracheostomy is very important. It involves checking the securement of the device every shift or more regularly to ensure it is in place, cleaning of the stoma site with 9% sodium chloride and proper drying at least once every day, artificial humidification is also done for patients, etc, suctioning is only done for those patients who can not clear their secretions on their own. Patients are often encouraged to cough and clear their own secretions. Suction is not given for more than 10 seconds to reduce chances of hypoxia, etc and if a patient has high oxygen requirements then pre-oxygenation must be done.

30:
Answer: D.   Measure blood pressure in upper extremities regularly

Explanation: Ssuperior vena cava syndrome is basically when there is a mechanical obstruction or compression of the superior vena cava due to various reasons like a tumor, enlarged lymph nodes, etc. The most common cause is a malignant disease. The primary treatment option is radiation therapy, while chemotherapy is the choice for patients who previously already received the maximum radiation dose. Surgical intervention is the choice only when the previous two treatments have failed. Nursing care includes various measures to relieve dyspnea like elevating the bed, providing oxygen, avoiding measurements of BP in upper extremities due to the presence of central venous access, assessment of radiation therapy side effects like skin changes, fatigue, dyspnea, etc, and side effects of chemotherapy like nausea, leukopenia, stomatitis, fatigue, anemia, etc. Nurses also teach the patient and his family about self care like use of mouth rinses, notifying increased temperature, etc, nurses must assess side effects of corticosteroids like weakness of involuntary muscles, mood swings, insomnia, etc. also easements for post operative coping by looking out for signs of depression, anxiety, and also pain must be done by the nurse.

31:
Answer: A.   Mutations in p53 are the most common genetic event related to cancer

Explanation: The p53 gene is a tumor suppressor gene and helps in the prevention of tumor formation normally. Any mutation in the gene will result in carcinogenesis. Li-Fraumeni syndrome, where only one functional copy of the gene is inherited predisposes the individual to cancer. Mutation in p53 is the most common genetic change associated with various cancers of the lung, breast, colon, etc. Various studies have shown that its mutation is linked to reduced survival rates in colorectal cancer.

32:
Answer: B.   Disclosure of your medical information to anyone other than medical staff in the hospital

Explanation: Patients including cancer survivors have a wide range of rights including those by the American hospital association (AHA), the national institute of health (NIH), the affordable care act (ACA), and the health insurance portability and accountability act (HIPAA). Under the federal law, the patient has various rights like access to medical records, your health information cannot be used for marketing or advertising purposes, you have the right to request changes to your medical records, etc. HIPAA gives you the right to control who may receive your medical records and what information they may receive. You also have the right to get insurance despite any pre-existing medical conditions.

33:
Answer: D.   Gram positive bacteria
Explanation: In the recent past various studies have established that gram positive bacteria are the most common organisms that lead to sepsis, which is due to the increased use of intravascular devices and pneumonia. Organisms like S. Aureus, S. Pyogens, E. Coli, etc are commonly isolated bacteria in sepsis. In normal bacteremia the erythrocytes and phagocytes eliminate the bacteria. However, sepsis causing bacteria evade this by the release of antioxidant enzymes, exopolymers, etc. Sepsis causing bacteria may directly infect the host and also release exotoxins or endotoxins, both of which cause various complications. Septic shock is due to bacterial endotoxin release. Cancer and its treatment often lead to decreased immunity in the patient, thus this host risk factor allows the sepsis causing bacteria to grow and leads to various complications like septic shock. Symptoms of septic shock include low blood pressure, fever, chills, an altered mental state and organ dysfunction, etc. Treatment includes the use of iv antibiotics, fluids, corticosteroids, etc.

34:
Answer: D.   Focusses on emotion
Explanation: The answer is "Focusses on emotion." This is an intrapsychic process-based coping skill because it focuses on the emotions that a person is feeling. By focusing on their emotions, they can better understand and deal with them.

35:
Answer: D. Gynecomastia

Explanation: Gynecomastia is the most prevalent side effect of diethylstilbestrol treatment for a patient with prostate cancer. This side effect is characterized by the enlargement of male breasts. Diethylstilbestrol can also cause other side effects, such as nausea, vomiting, and diarrhea.

36:
Answer: D. Bone

Explanation: Bone cancer is cancer that starts in the bone cells. Bone cancer can spread quickly to other parts of the body.

37:
Answer: B. Opioid drug use

Explanation: Nausea and vomiting are common in up to 70% of those patients with advanced cancer. It increases with an increase in disease severity. Nausea is the unpleasant feeling of the need to vomit. The causes of nausea and contains have to both be assessed. It can be due to various factors like chemical changes due to drugs like opioids, delayed gastric emptying due to medications like antidepressants, hepatomegaly, autonomic dysfunction; gastrointestinal obstructions; raised intracranial pressure; anxiety, etc. Treatment involves assessment of the likely cause, severity of symptoms, and use of non-pharmacological and pharmacological measures to manage nausea and vomiting. Various antiemetics used include metoclopramide, haloperidol, cyclizine, steroids like dexamethasone, 5HT3 receptor antagonists like ondansetron, etc. Non-pharmacological approaches such as Behavioural changes, acupuncture, etc.

38:
Answer: C. Provide the fastest relief to breakthrough pain according to research

Explanation: Many patients receiving end of life care for various reasons like cancer experience immense pain. Various options are available to provide pain relief and improve their quality of life. For those patients who experience breakthrough pain which involves periodic pain despite the use of analgesics according to a specific schedule, the FDA has approved and proven the efficacy of oral transmucosal fentanyl which provides the fastest relief for such pain. Breakthrough pain is usually idiopathic and its treatment provides an ease to the patient and allows improved social interactions and functioning.

39:
Answer: A.   Pancrelipase

Explanation: Whipple procedure involves the removal of the head of the pancreas, duodenum, gallbladder, and part of the bile duct. Due to this, the normal enzymes produced by the pancreas that aid in the digestion of food is lost. Hence, doctors prescribe pancreatic enzymes which have to be taken before food and will help in the normal digestion of proteins, carbohydrates, and fats. Other nutritional guidelines to follow include eating nutrient-dense food, avoiding fried and fatty food, eating small meals, etc.

40:
Answer: C.   Dysplastic Nevi

Explanation: Skin cancer is one the most common types of cancer. There are three major types of skin cancers- Melanoma, Basal cell carcinoma (BCC), and Squamous CEll Carcinoma (SCC). Both BCC and SCC are non-melanoma type cancers. Merkel cell tumors and dermatofibrosarcoma protuberans are other rare types of skin cancer. Malignant melanoma is a very aggressive cancer. Usually, skin cancers all start as precancerous lesions like- actinic keratosis, moles, or dysplastic nevi. Skin cancers can be caused for various reasons like immunosuppression, high exposure to radiation like UV radiation, tanning procedures, etc. Treatment for BCC and SCC usually involves surgical removal of tumor, while malignant melanoma requires more complicated treatment depending on its stage and spread including chemotherapy, radiation therapy, etc.

41:

Answer: A. **Severe diarrhea which may require medications like loperamide**

Explanation: Neratinib is used to treat cancer and it acts by interfering in the growth of cancer cells. The most common side effect of neratinib is diarrhea which may be severe and can lead to various complications like dehydration, hypotension, kidney failure, etc. Thus, often medication for diarrhea is given initially like loperamide, until the body gets used to the medication. Various side effects of the drug include diarrhea, confusion, dry skin, bladder pain, dry mouth, dizziness, thirst, etc. Some side effects do not require medical attention and decrease as the body gets used to the medication, while some require medical attention.

42:

Answer: A. **Cultural competence**

Explanation: A culturally competent nurse will aim to display politeness, knowledge of the patients' culture, and respect for the patients' beliefs. She will also be aware of her own cultural biases and be willing to learn about other cultures.

43:

Answer: C. **Confirmation of the diagnosis is done by colposcopic examination and biopsy**

Explanation: Cervical cancer is one of the most common malignancies found in women. It usually occurs in women above the age of 30 years and the HPV virus is one the most common causes of it.Hence HPV vaccine will help to provide protection against HPV-related cervical cancers. Screening helps in early diagnosis and usually involves pap smear and HPV testing. It is possible to get false positive and false negative with a Pap smear, and hence colposcopy examination and biopsy of any suspected lesion will help in the definitive diagnosis of cervical cancer.

44:

Answer: A. **To discontinue the administering of chemotherapeutic agent**

Explanation: If a patient experiences acute dyspnea, wheezing, hypotension, and throat and facial edema after intravenous injection of a chemotherapeutic agent, the nurse's first response should be to discontinue the infusion. This is because these symptoms may indicate anaphylactic shock, which is a potentially life-threatening condition. Other treatments may be necessary depending on the severity of the reaction.

45:
Answer: A.   Sepsis
Explanation: Sepsis after and during chemotherapy is a common side effect. Sepsis is basically when the body responds in a life-threatening manner to infection and can lead to tissue damage, organ failure, and death. Chemotherapy doesn't just kill cancer cells, but often good cells like the white blood cells are also killed off, leading to neutropenia. Due to this the body's ability to fight off infection decreases and the response to any bacteria, etc is heightened. Symptoms are usually a combination and include fever, body aches, diarrhea, breathing difficulties, skin changes, mental changes, etc. Signs include tachycardia, hypotension, altered respiratory rate, etc. Sepsis in cancer patients undergoing treatment is a medical emergency and requires immediate care.

46:
Answer: A.   Medication error
Explanation: All healthcare workers are expected to provide and uphold a level of standard care for patients. Failure to do so may result in severe problems and this negligence may result in Mahavir lawsuits also. Multiple missing errors may occur for various reasons. The errors include medication errors line wrong dosage, wrong time, wrong medicine, Failure to monitor vitals; Error in documentation; Failure to call a physician for timely assistance; Failing to update a patient's chart with changes in his or her progress; failure to feed the patient; etc. Out of these, medicine errors are the most common and one of the most dangerous errors to be made by a nurse. It is very important that the medicine name, dosage, timing, and route of administration be exactly as prescribed.

47:
Answer: A. Leukoreduced

Explanation: William may develop antibodies to the blood products he is receiving, necessitating the use of additional products such as leukoreduced blood products. Leukoreduced blood products have had the white blood cells removed, thereby reducing the risk of developing antibodies to these products.

48:
Answer: D. Cetirizine

Explanation: Drug-induced peripheral neuropathy occurs when the drug causes damage to the peripheral nervous system. The signs and symptoms may occur weeks or months after the use of the drug. There are various drugs that are known to cause peripheral neuropathy and hearing loss, and the pathophysiology associated is commonly damaged the dorsal root ganglia. All platinum chemotherapeutics are characterized by neuronopathic effects like the use of cisplatin and oxaliplatin. Vincristine is associated the greatest with the incidence of this and it is also seen with other vinca alkaloids like vinorelbine and vinblastine. Arsenic trioxide is used to treat APL often and a DIPN is a common noted side effect of it. Cetirizine is an antihistamine that has no effect on the peripheral nervous system.

49:
Answer: A. Specific suggestions

Explanation: PLISSIT is a model used to introduce a discussion about sex with the patient. P refers to permission where the patient is allowed to raise sexual concerns, LI refers to limited information about the sexual side effects of treatment to prevent inducing fear in the patient, and SS refers to specific suggestions given to the patient after a complete evaluation of the present problem like lubricants for vaginal dryness, and IT refers to intensive treatment which includes psychological counseling, sex therapy, biomedical approaches, etc.

50:

Answer: A.   Unrestrained and compulsive use of the drug for recreational purposes or despite negative consequences

Explanation: Opioids may be prescribed by doctors for pain management in various cases including chronic pains, cancer pain, post-surgery, etc and they may be given along with no opioids also. Due to the development of drug tolerance dosage may need to be increased for effective pain relief. When there is unrestrained and compulsive use of the drug for recreational purposes or despite negative consequences, even when it is not needed medically anymore, then the person is said to have an opioid addiction and it requires early intervention immediately.

51:

Answer: A.   Following religious and social practices that help deal with grief

Explanation: Grief is an emotional suffering experienced due to the loss of someone or something important to and loved by the person. The grieving process is highly personalized and everyone deals with it differently. People usually go through the five stages of grief which includes - denial, anger, bargaining, depression, and acceptance. It is important that the person grieves naturally and in a healthy manner. Use of medications and other substances for quick distraction and to numb the pain is strictly discouraged. Ignoring the grief is also discouraged. Patients must learn to accept their feelings, express them freely which may include crying, and learn to move ahead. Various religious customs like praying and social practices like therapy may help the patient through the grieving process. Isolation from others may worsen the situation due to unwanted thoughts and overthinking. Hence they should be engaged in social settings.

52:

Answer: D.   ' I might experience permanent hair loss '

Explanation: The patient might experience permanent hair loss. Radiation therapy can cause hair loss, usually temporary, but it's possible that some or all of the hair might not grow back.

53:

Answer: D.   Obstruction in the upper urinary tract

Explanation: The nurse suspects that the patient is experiencing an obstruction in the upper urinary tract. This can be caused by a tumor, scar tissue, or an enlarged prostate. The symptoms include difficulty urinating, pain in both flanks, and hyperkalemia.

54:

Answer: C.   Gemtuzumabozogamicin

Explanation: Jonas' recommended treatment is gemtuzumabozogamicin. This is a drug that specifically targets CD 33-positive cells, which are the cells that are most commonly found in acute myeloid leukemia. By targeting these cells, the drug can kill them and improve the patient's prognosis.

55:

Answer: D.   Commonly arises in response to a stimulus from the musculoskeletal system

Explanation: Nociceptive pain is caused by the triggering of nociceptors by various stimuli, whereas neuropathic pain arises due to damage to neurons. Features of nociceptive pain include- arising from the musculoskeletal system commonly, involves noxious stimuli triggering nociceptors. First line of management includes analgesics.

56:

Answer: A.   Is the second leading cause of cancer in women

Explanation: The average risk of an American woman developing breast cancer is 13%. It has been reported that breast cancer is the second leading cause of death in women who have cancer, with lung cancer being the first. There has been a decrease in overall female breast cancer related deaths over the last few decades which is said to be due to improved treatments, increased awareness, and better screening. Risk factors in women related to breast cancer include age, menopause, genetics, etc. A male breast cancer diagnosis is said to be quite rare.

57:

Answer: C.   Inflammatory breast cancer

Explanation: Multiple factors affect the prognosis of breast cancer. Regional lymph node spread, metastasis, tumors larger than 5 cm, negative estrogen receptor association, etc contribute to poor prognosis. Inflammatory breast cancer (IBC) is associated with a poor prognosis. It does not usually present as swollen lymph nodes and is not found in mammograms. They present with symptoms of breast tenderness and redness of more than 1/3rd breast, thickening or pitting of breast skin, swollen breast, inverted or retracted nipple, etc. IBC is more aggressive and usually presents with metastasis. It is more commonly seen in those younger than 40 years.

58:
Answer: B.   Increased intracranial pressure
Explanation: Increased intracranial pressure can be due to various reasons like tumors in the brain, metastatic cancers, etc. Radiation therapy of the brain may also cause an increase in intracranial pressure due to swelling of the brain caused by radiation. it may be right away (called acute increased ICP) or it can start later after radiation therapy has finished (called delayed increased ICP). Symptoms depend on the part of the brain that swells up and it may include poor memory, confusion, nausea, headache, behavior changes, nervous system problems like weakness in the legs and vision problems, etc. treatment for increased intracranial pressure may include medications and/or surgery.

59:
Answer: B.   Nonopioids are used first along with adjuvants and then opioid if needed

Explanation: Pain management for cancer-related pain at end of life is important to help provide ease for the patient and improve their quality of life. It is important to do pain assessment regularly to ensure that adequate pain management is provided to the patient. According to the WHO step-ladder pain management is advised where first nonopioids with/without adjuvants and then the addition of opioids for mild-moderate pain and lastly addition of opioids for moderate-severe pain. It is important to assess whether the patients have any contraindications for any medications and alter the medication as needed. For those with terminal illnesses, opioid analgesics are usually most effective. Intraspinal and epidural analgesics are both effective in relieving cancer pain in selected patients.

60:
Answer: D.   Increased fertility
Explanation: Various cancers like vulval, cervical, vaginal, etc may require pelvic radiation and/or chemotherapy. The sexual activity of a female is often affected during such treatments in various aspects. It may lead to early menopause as your ovaries are not working. This means infertility and has similar symptoms to normal menopause like hot flashes, mood swings, etc. This infertility may be temporary or permanent. The risk of which depends on radiation dosage, age, etc. Radiation can cause vaginal dryness, tenderness, scarring, fibrosis, and narrowing of the vagina. Various options for treatment of side effects of pelvic radiation and chemotherapy include vaginal reconstruction, pelvic floor exercises, dilators, etc.

61:
Answer: D.   It is considered the only treatment that the patient requires
Explanation: The generally accepted view is that when it comes to cancer treatment, surgery is the modal quality. This means that surgery is considered the most important and necessary treatment for cancer patients.

62:
Answer: D.   Diet

Explanation: Prostate cancer is the second leading cause of cancer-related deaths among men in the US. Various cancers have various risk factors with a few common risks. In relation to prostate cancer- age, family history, and race/ethnicity are strong risk factors, and genetics is also a known risk factor. There is a less-known risk association between prostate cancer and diet, obesity, smoking, etc. Age above 50 years, familial history of prostate cancer, African- American race, and genetic mutations of the BRCA1 Or BRCA2 genes are said to increase the risk of developing prostate cancer.

63:
Answer: B. Petechiae

Explanation: A person with acute myeloid leukemia may experience petechiae, which are small, red, or purple spots on the skin that are caused by bleeding. Other symptoms of this type of leukemia may include fatigue, shortness of breath, fever, and chest pain.

64:
Answer: C. Chances in skin appearance around stoma do not require special care

Explanation: A colostomy whether temporary or permanent has to be cared for properly. Colostomy care involves care of the skin around the stoma, the appliance, and the patient's mental health to prevent any complications related to it. The skin around the stoma must be the same as the abdomen, though it may at times be tender. Any swelling, rash, or redness may be indicative of an allergy or sensitivity and appropriate care must be taken. Various types of colostomy bags and appliances are available and the one most suitable for the patient is chosen. The 2-piece system is more long-lasting but needs the skill to use while the 1- piece system is simpler but must be changed every 3 days. Care includes emptying the bag when it is ½-⅓ full for ease of emptying, changing the appliance every 3-5 days, emptying the bag prior to chemotherapy, selecting the appropriate bag size for stoma, changing the bag in case of any leakage, etc.

65:
Answer: D. Dactinomycin

Explanation: Dactinomycin is a vesicant, meaning that it causes blisters. It is used as a chemotherapy drug to treat cancer.

66:
Answer: A.   Lung cancer
Explanation: Chemotherapy while used as a treatment modality has various long-term side effects. Hodgkin's lymphoma when treated using long-term chemotherapy with various alkylating agents like procarbazine, mechlorethamine, etc, like those used in MOPP chemotherapy, is known to have various side effects which include secondary malignancies. The risk for secondary malignancies further increases with the use of both chemotherapy and radiation. After chemotherapy alone, the most common second malignancy is lung cancer. Other second malignancies include non-HL and leukemias.

67:
Answer: A.   Pain control is not sufficient
Explanation: The nurse's suspicions are that the pain medication is not sufficient, as the patient is exhibiting behaviors that suggest they are in pain. This includes hyperventilation, sobbing, clenched fists, and inflexible lying.

68:
Answer: D.   Mismatched and unrelated donors are preferred
Explanation: When a bone marrow transplant is carried out and the donor immune cells attack the recipient's normal tissues, then it's called graft-vs-host disease (GVHD). It can either be acute or chronic depending on the pathophysiology. Acute GVHD mainly affects the skin and GIT, while chronic GVHD affects multiple systems like eyes, oral mucosa, lungs, skin, etc with signs of inflammation and fibrosis seen. Various preventive measures include sending 6/6 HLA matched and related donors, administration of various drugs like methotrexate, a calcineurin inhibitor, immunosuppressants like cyclophosphamide, and ex vivo or in vivo t-cell depletion methods. A number of other preventive measures are being studied for more effective use in GVHD like mesenchymal stromal cells, rituximab, and pentostatin.

69:
Answer: B. Repeating the same message in a different form
Explanation: Cancer education campaigns can focus on adults with low literacy rates by repeating the same message in a different form. This will help ensure that all individuals have the opportunity to learn about cancer and its prevention. Additionally, providing visuals or multimedia content may be helpful for those with low reading skills.

70:
Answer: C. Repeated attempts to insert 18 gauge needle
Explanation: Venous irritation is one of the complications associated with peripheral intravenous therapy. This can be due to the use of large gauge needles and repeated venous access attempts, due to extravasation of drugs, incorrect iv access placement, varied pH of the drug, etc. Venous irritation presents with symptoms of pain at the injection site and vein discoloration.

71:
Answer: A. Tissue biopsy
Explanation: CT scan may help in identifying possible lesions present in the lung that may not be detected by x-ray . Sputum cytology involves observing sputum under a microscope for abnormal cells. Both these methods are not definitive diagnostic methods as the changes observed may or may not actually be cancerous. However, the location of the lesion can be assessed with CT, and sputum cytology is useful in staging and treatment planning but may or may not be positive. Tissue biopsy involves the removal of abnormal cells from the doubtful area and careful analysis of the cells in the lab. A biopsy can be done in various ways like mediastinoscopy, needle biopsy, etc.

72:
Answer: D. Varicella zoster virus

Explanation: Infection is a side effect of hematopoietic stem cell transfer(HSCT) that needs to be taken care of in the short and long term also. The infection course after HSCT can be divided into three phases. The first is, during the conditioning to engraftment period which ranges from 5-30 days sending on the type of transplant. The second is engraftment to post-transplant day 100 during which infection with cytomegalovirus is the most likely, followed by few herpes viruses like Epstein Barr virus and invasive mold infections also. The third is more than 100 days post-transplant, in the absence of graft-versus-host-disease, during which infection with varicella zoster virus, PCP, and pneumococcal infection may occur. Prophylactic use of trimethoprim/sulfamethoxazole and acyclovir significantly decreases the risk of infection with PCP and herpes-virus infections, respectively.

73:
Answer: C. Needle repositioning and coughing of patient

Explanation: A port or implanted venous access device consists of a reservoir placed under the skin and a hollow tube placed in a vein. It helps establish a central line for those who need repeated intravenous access. Access is achieved by the insertion of a needle into the tube. Once a syringe is inserted, then pull back on the syringe is done to check for blood return. In case of no blood return but the flushing is normal, then the first thing to do is reposition the needle and ask the patient to cough or change position slightly to change intrathoracic pressure. If this does not work then re-accessing of port with the new needle may be done, then if the problem persists declotting, dye study, x-rays, or ultrasounds may be done to solve the issue.

74:
Answer: C. It provides a clear idea about the care and surveillance after treatment

Explanation: The most significant advantage of a survivorship care plan is that it provides a clear idea about the care and surveillance after treatment. This allows for better communication between the patient, health care professionals, and loved ones. Additionally, it helps to ensure that any potential late effects of cancer treatment are identified and managed proactively.

75:
Answer: B.   **Endometrial**

Explanation: Rosie's postmenopausal bleeding could be a result of uterine cancer. Uterine cancer is the most common cancer in women, and it is most likely to occur in women who are over 60 and obese. Rosie also has diabetes, which increases her risk of developing uterine cancer.

76:
Answer: C.   **Setting a comfortable bedroom temperature**

Explanation: A comfortable bedroom temperature would help reduce sleep disturbances. The temperature has been shown to be one of the most important factors in determining human sleep quality.

77:
Answer: B.   **Has lower rates of success than allograft transplantation**

Explanation: Autograft transplantation is a process where the patient's healthy stem cells are collected from bone marrow prior to treatment with chemotherapy or radiation, and then given back to the patient after treatment. It helps in the replacement of patients' stem cells that may be damaged during radiation or chemotherapy. It is commonly used to treat leukemia and lymphoma. It requires the presence of healthy bone marrow and hence cannot be done in patients with diseases like aplastic anemia. It has a lower infection rate and GVHD is not an issue as patients' own stem cells are being used, thus leading to better success rates than allograft transplantation.

78:
Answer: D.   **Neutropenia occurs after 22 to 28 days of completion**

Explanation: The nurse will give the patient instructions on how to take temozolomide and what adverse effects to watch for. The patient should take the medication exactly as prescribed. If vomiting occurs, they should take the medication with a small amount of water and then drink plenty of fluids. The patient should also watch for signs of infection and report any symptoms to the healthcare provider. Temozolomide can cause neutropenia (low white blood cell count), so the patient will need to be monitored for this side effect. They may need to have their blood counts checked regularly while taking the medication.

79:
Answer: D. **Making the patient resume work immediately after treatment**

Explanation: Nurses have an important role in the treatment and management of cancer patients. Nursing care involves assessment, diagnosis, planning, implementation, and evaluation. For cancer patients focus is on ensuring proper treatment plan and execution, supportive care for various symptoms like fatigue, nausea, hair loss, etc, and other mental and social issues faced by the patient. The involvement of family and friends in the care plan is important to provide the patient with peer support and care. The patient and his support system must be informed about the diagnosis, treatment, and progress of the patient regularly. Methods to introduce the patient back into his normal life post successful treatment are also important. The patient must not be rushed to get back to his/her previous life as cancer and its treatment comes with a wide array of mental, physical, social, and spiritual changes that need to be dealt with in a healthy manner.

80:
Answer: D. **Trespassing**

Explanation: A nurse's license may be revoked due to various reasons and these vary from state to state in the US. It is important to know what is classified as a misdemeanor in your state as this usually results in sanctions and not revocation.

However there are certain felonies for almost sure-shot revocation of license and these include violation of preexisting suspension/probation, use of the fake license, abusing a patient, kidnapping, murder, etc. Various misdemeanors that may result in suspension but not felony usually include alcohol abuse, charting errors, trespassing, criminal conviction, etc. Suspension results in various things like penalty fines, educational remediation, imposing monitoring, etc.

81:
Answer: D.   Iv morphine

Explanation: Metastatic cancer may lead to the presence of malignant cells in the pleural fluid which is a very disabling condition. It leads to a huge negative impact on patients' quality of life. Dyspnea is a common symptom patients present with. Sometimes cough, chest pain, etc may also be present. Lung and breast cancer are the most common metastatic cancers related to this. Treatment approaches include :
- repeated thoracentesis where small catheters are used and have a high chance of recurrence; pleurodesis with agents like talc, bleomycin, etc;
- Video assisted thoracic surgery (VATS) talc poudrage;
- IPC are semi- implantable devices that make use of a vacuum at home to drain pleural effusions;

82:
Answer: B.   Laryngeal cancer

Explanation: Cancers of the larynx (voice box) can be caused by excessive use of smokeless tobacco and alcohol. These cancers arise from the cells that line the larynx. They can be very aggressive and can spread to other parts of the body, such as the lungs or brain.

83:
Answer: C.   Self reporting

Explanation: The patient's major source of information for determining the amount of pain is self-reporting. This means that the patient is usually the best source of information about the level of pain they are experiencing. Physicians and other healthcare providers may ask patients to rate their pain on a scale of 1 to 10, for example, to help determine the appropriate treatment.

84:
Answer: D. 2400

Explanation: Weight loss is common amongst cancer patients and is often referred to as cachexia which has signs and symptoms of fatigue, loss of appetite, increased metabolism, etc. Cancer or its treatment-related side effects can lead to weight loss. Ensuring the weight of the patient is normal and not underweight includes proper calorie intake according to the patient's weight and physical activity. In the current case for a patient to maintain weight, multiply it by 13 (if you don't exercise at all), 15 (if you exercise a few times weekly), or 18 (if you exercise five days or more a week). In cancer patients, the disease and treatment increase the patient's metabolism and exerts the patients as equal to high levels of activity and there is a requirement for higher calorie intake to maintain weight, hence the patient's current weight (135) can be multiplied by 18, so here the calorie intake will be 18 x 135 = 2430 or roughly 2400 calories.

85:
Answer: A. Secondary leukemia

Explanation: Cyclophosphamide is a type of chemotherapy that is used to treat various types of cancer. While it is an effective treatment for many patients, it can also cause a number of side effects. One possible side effect is secondary leukemia, which is a form of blood cancer that can develop after treatment with cyclophosphamide. Secondary leukemia can cause bruising and fatigue, among other symptoms. Therefore, it appears that secondary leukemia may be the culprit for Michelle's recent symptoms.

86:
Answer: B. Refusing any sort of religious practices within hospital premises

Explanation: Practices' basic needs should be fulfilled during their diagnosis and treatment also. This includes their spiritual needs. It is a delicate matter and must be approached respectfully. Nurses should openly communicate about the spiritual needs of the patient and respect their choices. Various spiritual practices may be performed by the patient in the hospital as long as it is not causing harm to the patient or anyone else. Offering spiritual assistance includes arranging meetings with their spiritual leaders to seek blessings, etc. Refusal to discuss or fulfill the spiritual needs of the patient affects the treatment outcome and disease prognosis, and hence must be respectfully addressed as part of patient care and treatment.

87:
Answer: A.   **Reiki therapy**

Explanation: Reiki therapy is the most appropriate integrative modality for a patient with pain and a platelet count of 12000/mm Reiki is a form of energy healing that is used to restore balance and alignment within the body. It can be used to treat a variety of conditions, including pain, and is gentle and calming, making it an ideal choice for patients who are anxious or stressed.

88:
Answer: D.   **Survivor Guilt**

Explanation: When Michelle says "I was always the difficult kid," she may be expressing survivor guilt. Survivor guilt is a feeling of guilt that may be experienced by someone who has survived a traumatic event while others have not. This may lead to feelings of self-blame or regret for being alive while others have died.

89:
Answer: D.   **Neighbours**

Explanation: Social dysfunction is common in cancer survivors and patients. They have fear of recurrence, anxiety, guilt, spiritual concerns, financial stress, etc. It is important that their healthcare providers and social circle are able to identify such signs and symptoms at the earliest like substance abuse, suicidal behavior, depression, etc. Psychosocial issues faced by the cancer survivor need to be addressed and treated. Treatment may include support groups, professional counseling, family counseling, spiritual practices, prescription of certain medications like antidepressants, etc. There is a 10-15% increase in the risk of relationships and hence all his relations being affected by this including family, friends, employer, etc may need to be involved in the process of the patient adjusting back to normal life. Neighbors unless part of the patient's close social circle does not need to be involved in this process specifically.

90:
Answer: B.   Cisplatin is the first drug of choice
Explanation: Cancer patients have a 5-7 times increased risk for Thromboembolic disease. In cancer patients, the tumor may compress veins and lead to venous stasis and further thrombosis. An arterial thrombus may occur due to systemic hypercoagulation induced by several secreted factors from cancer cells and chemotherapeutic agents like cisplatin, VEGF inhibitors, etc. Other severe manifestations of the procoagulant state in cancer patients are disseminated intravascular coagulation (DIC) and thrombotic microangiopathy (TMA). Thromboembolic disease is three times more commonly seen in non-cancer people and contributes to mortality and morbidity. Risk factors for this include older age, female sex, black race, presence of comorbid conditions, and hospitalization.

91:
 Answer: D.   Assess the patient need to define the problem

Explanation: The first step in utilizing evidence-based practices in a cancer care setting is to assess the patient's needs and define the problem. This involves gathering information about the patient's symptoms, diagnosis, and treatment history. The goal is to identify any gaps between the patient's current care and the best available evidence. Once the problem is defined, interventions can be selected and implemented that have the greatest potential to improve patient outcomes.

92:
**Answer: A.	Pouch Leakage**
Explanation: Skin irritation around the stoma after ileostomy is usually due to leakage from the ostomy pouch. This leakage causes the contents of the pouch to get under the adhesive and contact the skin. The leakage can be due to uneven skin surrounding the stoma, change in stoma shape/ size which occurs naturally, diet alterations that lead to unexpected filling of the bag, ballooning, pancaking, etc. To check this it's important to remove the adhesive and check the back of it for signs of any urine or feces that may have caused irritation. Changes in periosteal skin appearance can also be due to allergy, infection, etc, and hence the exact cause must be determined and treated as needed.

93:
Answer: B. Methotrexate
Explanation: Methotrexate is a chemotherapy agent and immuno-suppressant. Cancers treated by it include breast cancer, leukemia, and lung cancer. Folate is needed in the process of DNA synthesis and methotrexate is an antifolate agent which acts by inhibiting dihydrofolate reductase thus causing cancer cell death. It is administered either by injection or orally. Common side effects include liver damage, nausea, tiredness, low WBC count, increased infection risks. This also leads to abortions in pregnant women.

94:
**Answer: C.	Contact a representative of the patient to get consent**

Explanation: Consent is basically a legal concept based on the idea that adults of sound minds have the right to make informed decisions for themselves. However, there are various scenarios in the medical setup where obtaining informed consent from the patient may not be possible. This includes patients who have unmanaged mental illnesses, comatose patients, drowsy patients, patients who are disoriented due to severity of pain/disease, etc. Informed consents require the doctor to clearly explain the procedure to the patient inappropriate words, however often in emergencies this is shortened and patients may not be in a state to give immediate, well-informed consents. In such cases, it is vital to immediately contact a representative of the patient and obtain consent first. If the representative is not reachable, delays in the medical intervention will result in harm to the patient. Here the doctor may declare a medical emergency and perform surgery. The doctor must take the most well thought and well-informed decision in such situations.

95:
Answer: D. Sustained fever which does not improve with paracetamol consumption also

Explanation: Biologic therapies cause various side effects when used which need to be managed as and when they appear. Interleukin is known to cause flu-like symptoms including chills, fever, body aches, etc. Proper symptomatic management must be followed. General fever is a side effect that is easily managed with paracetamol, but if not manageable and is continuously present, then further investigations must be done to rule out any severe effects. Fatigue or extreme tiredness is very common while undergoing biological agent therapy which usually goes away once treatment is done but for some people may be chronic. Some people experience allergic reactions to the medications like coughing, chest pain, skin rash, etc, and these symptoms are managed as they appear and may require dose alteration if severe. Weight loss or weight gain are also side effects of biological agent therapy.

96:
Answer: A. Demonstrates the spread to the liver

Explanation: The tumor cells of pancreatic invasive ductal adenocarcinoma can spread (metastasize) to other parts of the body, most commonly the liver.

97:

Answer: A.   The patient must have an adequate performance status

Explanation: The most significant criterion for choosing patients for a phase 2 clinical trial is the patient's performance status. Patients who are unable to complete the trial's required activities or who are at risk of death are typically not selected for phase 2 trials. In addition, patients who have not responded to previous treatments may also be excluded from phase 2 trials.

98:

Answer: D.   Stereotyping patients to ensure better and quicker treatment

Explanation: Cultural differences and minorities must be understood and respected during patient care. Nurses have to be educated on the various effects of culture and race on patient diagnosis and treatment planning. Verbal and non-verbal commission are different for different cultures and must be respected, for example, certain cultures may be more open and have less body spacing, while some accept more distance and lesser contact. Language may pose a barrier and hence requirements for translated material and a translator must be arranged for as needed. Nurses must not stereotype, discriminate, disregard, or neglect patients based on their culture or race. Culturally and racially aware communication and treatment are most important.

99:

Answer: C.   Methotrexate

Explanation: Various drugs are given to a cancer patient during chemotherapy that is meant to target the cancer cells but unfortunately they do have few negative effects on other cells. The liver is one such organ in the body that may get adversely affected due to long term use of certain medications in cancer patients. Out of the mentioned drugs, methotrexate is the drug most likely to lead to fatty liver, liver fibrosis, and cirrhosis on long term use. It is known to cause serum aminotransferase elevations. With long term, low-to-moderate dose methotrexate therapy, elevations in serum ALT or AST is seen in about 15% to 50% of the patients which is usually of low-to-moderate risk. Hence those on long term chemotherapy are advised to get regular follow-ups to assess any side effects that may appear due to treatment.

100:
Answer: B.   Demerol

Explanation: Various drugs can be used to treat neuropathic pain in cancer patients. Pharmacological agents used in these cases include opioids, non-opioids, and adjuvants. Adjuvants are those that are not primarily indicated for pain but have analgesic properties, and they are the first choice in such cases. Adjuvants include tricyclic antidepressants and anticonvulsants like Gabapentin, pregabalin, duloxetine, amitriptyline, venlafaxine, etc. Along with adjuvants, opioids or non-opioids may be given like codeine, acetaminophen, etc. Other drugs like ketamine which is an NMDA antagonist can also be used. Non-pharmacological management of pain is also commonly used. Meperidine (Demerol) is contraindicated for chronic pain treatment in cancer patients because it may cause CNS toxicity, with mood swings coming experienced.

101:
Answer: A.   MRI

Explanation: Various tumors in the body may metastasize and reach the brain causing changes in functions of the brain and surrounding tissues due to tumor pressure on tissues. The symptoms presented vary depending on which part of the brain is affected, the size of the tumor, etc. Common symptoms of brain metastasis include - headache, nausea, memory issues, weakness, behavior changes, vision changes. Magnetic resonance imaging (MRI) is commonly used to help diagnose brain metastases in which a dye may be injected through a vein in your arm during your MRI study. Specialized MRI scans including functional MRI, perfusion MRI and magnetic resonance spectroscopy — may help your doctor evaluate the tumor and plan treatment. Other diagnostic aids like CT scan, Pet scan, biopsy, etc may also be employed.

102:
Answer: D.   Amitriptyline

Explanation: Amitriptyline is an effective treatment for severe pain caused by postherpetic neuropathy. Amitriptyline is a tricyclic antidepressant that blocks nerve impulses, which helps to relieve pain.

103:
Answer: D.   **Cancer antigen 125 in the blood is a definitive diagnostic tool for it**

Explanation: Ovarian cancer is usually seen in older women of ages 60 years. The early disease may present no symptoms, as the disease progresses it presents various symptoms including abdominal bloating, abnormal fullness, increased urination, difficulty eating, and back pain. Risk factors include a family history of ovarian cancer, obesity, older age, genetic mutations like BRCA1 and BRCA2, hormone therapy use, and endometriosis. Various diagnostic tools include transvaginal ultrasound, abdominal and pelvic CT, blood CA-125 levels, and biopsy. A biopsy is the only definitive diagnostic tool. Transvaginal ultrasound cannot detect small tumors and CA-125 blood levels are affected by menstruation and uterine fibroids also.

104:
Answer: B.   Constipation

Explanation: 5-HT3 antagonists are drugs commonly used to control nausea and vomiting caused by chemotherapy, radiation therapy, IBS, etc. They act by blocking serotonin binding to 5-HT3 receptors and hence slow gut motility and delay the passing of food through the small intestine. This slowing of bowel movements may lead to constipation in patients, along with abdominal pain, and headaches.

105:
Answer: D.   Stopping aspirin, and taking opioids regularly

Explanation: Cancer pain is a huge issue in cancer patients and it is said that inadequate pain management in such cases may also be the cause of death. The world health organization suggested a ladder method for treatment of cancer pain which includes three steps- (1) initial administration of non-opioids (like NSAIDS and COX-2 inhibitors) and proceeding to the next step if pain persists; (2) administration of opioids for mild to moderate pain along with non-opioids and proceeding to next step if pain persists; (3) administration of opioids for moderate to severe pain along with non-opioids and titrate till adequate pain control is achieved. When both non-opioids and opioids are given, and the limit for non-opioids is reached, ex->4g/day for paracetamol, then pure opioid therapy is started. Usually, opioids already are given with acetaminophen, hence additional use of it is not needed when taking opioids in these cases.

106:
Answer: C.   Avoiding tobacco products

Explanation: The easiest way to cure cancer is to prevent it. Various primary preventive measures can be followed which will lower the risk of getting cancer. These include healthy lifestyle choices like avoiding tobacco products, following a nutritional diet, regular physical activity, protection from uv rays, etc. Healthy environments must also be maintained and encouraged like green surroundings, smoke-free areas, etc. Pap smears and breast examinations help with early diagnosis and not prevention of cancer.

107:
Answer: C.   Poor nutrition has not affect on alopecia

Explanation: Hair loss is a well-known side effect of cacner tretament with chemotherapy and radiation therapy and is known as alopecia. It affects hair all over the body in chemotherapy and hair in the area where radiation is aimed. A few chemotherapeutic drugs that cause hair loss are altretamine, carboplatin and cisplatin. Hormonal therapy with a few drugs like anastrozole, fulvestrant, etc may cause thinning of hair and hair loss. The risk for alopecia is more when the patient has a poor nutritional status and many drugs are used for cancer treatment. Management of this side effect included the use of cooling caps, scalp cryotherapy, minoxidil drug applied to the scalp. Care of hair during cancer treatment to prevent/decrease alopecia includes washing hair gently and less often, using mild shampoos, using silk pillow cases, avoiding any heat treatments, and avoiding ponytails. A scarf or wig can be worn by the patient if he/she prefers. Alopecia is temporary and hair regrows after cancer treatment is stopped.

108:
Answer: B.   **Female-to-male donation**
Explanation: Acute graft versus host disease is a reaction of the donor's immune cells against the host tissue. Organs mainly affected are the skin, liver, and GI tract. Symptoms include skin rash, abdominal cramps, and hepatitis. The risk of acute graft versus host disease increases with the use of unrelated donors, older age of the donor, certain conditioning regimens, opposite gender donor and recipient, and multiparous female donor.

109:
Answer: C.   **Use non-acetone nail polish remover**
Explanation: Chemotherapy with drugs like paclitaxel may lead to changes in the nails. Nails become weaker, brittle, are more likely to peel off, and indentation on nails is seen. While getting professional manicures during chemotherapy, it is suggested to advise the parlor incharge to be gentle and use non-acetone nail polish remover as it is less drying. Gentle moisturizers can be used to hydrate the skin of the hands and nails. Avoiding nail extensions is advised as they can be harsh on the nails.

110:

Answer: A.   Prealbumin

Explanation: A test commonly used to evaluate acute changes in nutritional status is prealbumin. This measures the level of a protein in the blood that is released from the liver. It is often used to monitor the dietary status of patients with cachexia, which is a condition characterized by weight loss and muscle wasting. The most frequently observed change in prealbumin levels is a decrease in those levels.

111:
Answer: C.   Usage of sunscreen

Explanation: Sunscreen usage is the principal method of cancer prevention. Sunscreen use can help reduce the risk of developing skin cancer, including melanoma. Sunscreen should be applied regularly and liberally to all exposed skin, especially during periods of sun exposure.

112:
Answer: B.   The infusion of the medication has to be stopped

Explanation: If a patient complains of urticaria and itching after receiving paclitaxel, the nurse will stop the infusion of the medication. Urticaria and itching are potential side effects of paclitaxel, so it is important to stop the infusion if these symptoms occur.

113:
Answer: A.   Diet high in fibers

Explanation: A diet high in fibers and low in fat will help prevent colorectal cancer. Family history of this in first-degree relatives or others will increase the risk. Higher amounts of red meat and processed food will put the person at risk for the disease. Rare inherited diseases like Lynch syndrome, Gardner syndrome, and familial adenomatous polyposis may lead to colorectal cancer. Inflammatory bowel diseases like Crohn's disease also may lead to this. Prevention includes eating nutritious foods, avoiding smoking, maybe use of NSAIDS, and regular screening to detect and treat precancerous lesions.

114:
Answer: D.   Use personal protective equipment

Explanation: Exposure to hazardous drugs have acute and chronic effects ranging from nausea and vomiting to cancer and reproductive issues. During dialysis, it's important to ensure the safety of the healthcare workers against these possible negative effects. Hence all medications being used by the patient must be conveyed to the doctors and nurses administering the dialysis procedure. The dialysis staff must be informed and trained to deal with hazardous medication prior to treating such patients. To best ensure the safety of all those involved, the use of various personal protective measures like double gloving can be followed.

115:
Answer: D.   Include vaccination of all premenopausal women
Explanation: The quadrivalent human papillomavirus vaccine (gardasil) protects against infection from HPV 6,11,16 and 8 which also contributes to 70% of cervical cancers. Under the immunization program, the vaccine is currently administered to females between 9-26 years of age. This vaccine can also be used in boys of ages 9-26 to prevent anal cancer and genital warts. This vaccine does not eliminate the need for a PAP smear and does not protect against STDs. This vaccine will NOT cure active HPV infection or active genital warts/HPV-related cancers.

116:
Answer: C.   Mortality rates are higher in black women

Explanation: Breast cancer is a common cancer and is the most common cause of cancer related deaths in women. Racial disparities amongst whites and African-Americans when it comes to breast cancer are quite prevalent. The overall incidence of breast cancer is now equal amongst both races now compared to the past when it was more common among whites. Triple negative breast cancer and inflammatory breast cancer however have a higher incidence among African Americans. Lack of screening amongst African Americans results in a diagnosis of more advanced-stage cancers. Aggressive cancers at a young age are more common in African Americans. Due to the lower socioeconomic status commonly associated with African Americans, they also have a lower survival rate and increased mortality due to breast cancer. It's important to note that whites also experience poverty and its effects on cancer treatment and diagnosis.

118:
Answer: A. 123 mg.
Explanation: Body surface area is essential for the administration of certain drugs. Various formulas are present to calculate the BSA but the most common is the Mosteller Equation: BSA (m2) = square root ([Height(cm) x Weight(kg)]/ 3600
The BSA IS then multiplied by the dose of 70 mg to get the total drug dosage.

119:
Answer: A. Provide a non-stimulating laxative
Explanation: If Richard is experiencing watery stools, lower abdominal pain, and a rectal issue, it is likely that he is suffering from an advanced stage of lung cancer that has progressed to the point of causing complications. In this case, the nurse should provide a non-stimulating laxative to help Richard alleviate his symptoms.

120:
Answer: C. Anaesthetic mouth rinses were given and no spicy food was advised

Explanation: Oral mucositis can be very painful and it affects the patient's quality of life and food intake. It involves erythema, erosions, and ulcers which can be very painful. These lesions usually disappear within 2-4 weeks post-chemotherapy. Management of chemotherapy-induced mucositis involves pain management with anesthetic mouth rinses, nutritional support to ensure the patient gets enough nutrients and if needed gastrostomy tube is placed, avoiding triggering foods like spicy food, oral decontamination measures to prevent infection of lesions, and management of any bleeding of lesions if present.

121:
Answer: D. Continue administration of same asparaginase formulation
Explanation: Asparaginase is commonly used to treat acute lymphoblastic leukemia but its complications include hypersensitivity reactions which limit its use. Hypersensitivity reactions may be clinical or subclinical. Clinical allergic reaction to asparaginase as seen in this patient is due to the formation of anti-asparaginase antibodies and thus continuing the same formulation will not work even with the use of premedications, which will only prevent the symptoms. Administration of asparaginase levels is important to know the amount of drug in the body. Vitals must also be monitored as hypersensitivity reactions can manifest symptoms ranging from pruritus, itchy eyes, etc to breathing difficulties, decreased heart rate, etc. Alternative asparaginase formulations may be administered, as Erwinia asparaginase is antigenically distinct from E. coli-derived or peg- asparaginase. Administration of emergency medications like antihistamines, adrenaline, etc to treat the symptoms is important to prevent them from worsening, and continued iv saline to help flush out the drug. As the patient has known allergies it's important to have tested for asparaginase allergy prior to starting treatment and premedication with steroids or antihistamines should have been done.

122:
Answer: A. Constipation
Explanation: The most prevalent palonosetron side effect is constipation. This occurs in about 9% of people who take the medication. Other common side effects include headache, diarrhea, and nausea.

123:
Answer: C.   Mutation affecting only one or few nucleotides in a gene sequence

Explanation: Proto-oncogenes are normal genes in the cell that when mutated become oncogenes, i.e. cause cancer development. Ras is a proto-oncogene that encodes for an intracellular signal-transduction protein, which means it affects cell growth. Point mutation occurs in the Ras gene which means one or few of the nucleotides in the gene sequence are altered and this in turn leads to uncontrolled growth-promoting signals. Ras mutations are the cause of most types of pancreatic cancers and other cancers of the lung, and colon.

124:
Answer: D.   GI tract

Explanation: Radiation effect on the tissue depends on the amount and duration of exposure to radiation during therapy. Tissues with cells that get rapidly replaced are most affected by radiation and show early signs of cell destruction which include bone marrow mainly, GIT lining, and skin which manifest as skin erythema, neutropenia, and GI disturbances. Other slow-growing tissues like the brain require high doses and longer durations of radiation to undergo tissue changes and cell destruction. Tissue damage caused due to radiation is mainly due to cell depletion, inability to reproduce, decreased immunity to infections, etc.

125:
Answer: D.   Differentiation between breast and lung cancer

Explanation: Fatigue is a common side effect of cancer and its treatment. It can be assessed using various measures like Brief Fatigue Inventory, Fatigue Scale Adolescent, and Functional assessment of cancer therapy-General. The assessment of fatigue is useful to predict disease prognosis as extreme fatigue due to disease process alone is suggestive of poor prognosis. Cancer treatment is also planned and modified according to cancer fatigue experienced by. Admission into clinical trials for cancer also includes evaluation of various categories like cancer stage, drugs being used by patient, activity performance which is affected by cancer fatigue scores, etc. Hence admission into clinical trials requires fatigue assessment in cancer patients.

126:
Answer: A. **Most commonly associated with breast cancer and those who got axillary lymph node radiation/resection.**

Explanation: Lymphedema secondary to cancer treatment is a common occurrence and is said to have major negative effects on quality of life. While cancer infiltration into lymph nodes may itself cause lymphedema, a treatment that involves radiation/resection of axillary lymph nodes is said to lead to upper limb lymphedema. Various contributing factors include weight gain, injury to the arm, and lack of information about lymphedema. It is more commonly seen in women who undergo breast cancer treatment. Management and prevention of these precipitating factors are possible to a certain extent. Treatment done is usually complete or complex decongestive therapy (CDT) which includes compressions, skincare, manual lymph drainage, and exercise. Intermittent pneumatic compression is also often added to CDT.

127:
Answer: D. **Final approval of treatment plan**

Explanation: Nursing scope basically refers to the range of roles, functions, responsibilities, and activities that registered nurses are educated and authorized to perform. The scope of oncology nurses includes various responsibilities and functions like care of the patient through administration of doctor-approved treatment plans including chemotherapy, palliative care, patient education about the disease and treatment plan ,coordination of care between various departments of the hospital, advocate for cancer patients needs and rehabilitation of the patient. While nurses are allowed to administer certain medications for alleviating various symptoms, the final treatment plan carried out must be approved by a doctor with the patient/patient's family's approval.

128:
Answer: A.   5-fluorouracil
Explanation: 5-fluorouracil is a medication commonly used during chemotherapy and is hazardous. Doctors are unsure about whether semen or vaginal discharge contains chemotherapy drugs. Hence it is advised that patients being treated with chemotherapy use barrier protection like condoms, femidoms, etc to protect his/her sexual partner. This is advised only during treatment and for a week post treatment, after which it is not necessary.

129:
Answer: B.   Partial nephrectomy
Explanation: Surgical treatment of kidney cancer depends on the size and spread of the kidney. Stage 1 renal cancer usually means a tumor of less than 4 cm in size with no lymph node involvement or spread. Partial nephrectomy either laparoscopic or conventionally is advised in such cases and is proven to be effective as a treatment method. It helps in preserving the remaining unaffected kidney tissue thus allowing better recovery in case another kidney gets affected in the future or has poor renal functioning. Laparoscopic partial nephrectomy is said to be better as it is less invasive and recovery is quicker. Radical surgery involving removal of complete kidney and/or lymph nodes and/or adrenal gland possess higher risks for such patients with comorbid conditions.

130:
Answer: B.   Review the patient's medical report
Explanation: A patient's medical report would indicate whether or not the patient has a clotting disorder that is causing their abnormal bleeding. If the patient does have a clotting disorder, the nurse should provide intervention to treat the clotting disorder.

131:
Answer: D.   Emetine
Explanation: Nausea and vomiting due to cancer treatment are very common and the types are- acute, chronic, delayed, breakthrough, anticipatory and refractory. It is more commonly associated with chemotherapy. Measures to prevent and reduce this include pharmacological and nonpharmacological methods. Drugs used include dopamine receptor antagonists like chlorpromazine and metoclopramide, Serotonin receptor antagonists like ondansetron, corticosteroid like dexamethasone, and benzodiazepines like lorazepam. Non-pharmacological management includes acupuncture, music therapy, and dietary measures like eating smaller meals and avoiding fast foods. Both drugs and other methods can be combined for better effect. Emetine is a drug that induces vomiting and is commonly used as an antiprotozoal drug.

132:
Answer: A.   The linear accelerator is used for brachytherapy
Explanation: Radiation therapy involves the use of high intensity energy to kill cancer cells by causing damage to their DNA. It can be used as a primary, neoadjuvant, or adjuvant treatment of cancer. The two types are external radiation which uses a linear accelerator to deliver high beams of radiation and internal radiation where radioisotopes are used to internally provide radiation that targets cancer cells. Radioactive iodine is a common radioisotope used to treat thyroid cancer. Specific doses of radiation are administered to the patient which are measured in grays or centigrams.

133:

Answer: A.   Fluconazole

Explanation: Fluconazole is a medication that is used to treat infections caused by fungus. It is effective in treating oral erythema, white patches on the palate, xerostomia, and a lumpy sensation while swallowing.

134:
Answer: D.   Breast examinations by the doctor

Explanation: Women at high risk for breast cancer may be advised to take prescription drugs tamoxifen and raloxifene. Post-menopausal hormones both estrogen and estrogen-plus-progestin increase the risk of cancer. Smoking is said to increase the risk of 15 types of cancers including breast cancer. Breast examinations, while useful for early detection of breast cancer, will not help reduce the risk of its occurrence in any way.

135:
Answer: A.   Radiation dermatitis

Explanation: Radiation therapy involves the administration of high-intensity energy to the patient for various durations and in varying doses. This radiation may have various side effects which can be seen during the early stages of treatment or later. Early side effects often include fatigue and skin changes, GI disturbances, and bone marrow changes. Late side effects may occur months or years after radiation in any part of the body exposed to radiation like thicker skin over the breast, and inflammation of the lungs (radiation pneumonitis). Early skin changes seen include swollen skin, erythema, and itchy, flaky skin which is called radiation dermatitis. Other early effects were seen depending on the body part exposed to radiation and may include hair loss, and mouth changes.

136:
Answer: A.   To Sit upright most of the time

Explanation: The nurse will typically tell the patient to avoid inserting anything into the vagina for four weeks following a loop electrosurgical excision procedure. This includes avoiding sexual intercourse, tampons, and douching. This is to ensure that the area heals properly and does not become infected.

137:
Answer: B. Precancerous abnormal cells without spread to other tissues

Explanation: Carcinoma in situ basically refers to abnormal cells found in the place where they are originally formed without spreading to other tissues. There is a debate about whether to classify this as cancer or precancerous cells. Often it is referred to as stage 0 cancer and treatment options include laser, surgical removal of cancer cells, etc, which are said to be usually successful due to the non-invasive nature of the diagnosis. An example of carcinoma in situ is ductal carcinoma in situ which is said to be an early form of breast cancer and treatment usually involves surgery and radiation/hormonal therapy.

138:
Answer: A. IV calcium chlorate or gluconate

Explanation: Due to the history of acute myeloid leukemia and current chemotherapy, and the signs and symptoms presented by the patient means that he likely has tumor lysis syndrome (TLS). The rapid breakdown of tumor cells due to chemotherapy leads to hyperuricemia, hyperkalemia, hyperphosphatemia and hypocalcemia with various symptoms including urinary retention, muscle spasm, and other serious conditions like cardiac arrhythmia, hypotension. Treatment is done immediately when suspected as this is a life threatening condition. Hyperkalemia is the most important condition to be treated in such cases, which includes cardiac monitoring, nephrology consultation and hemodialysis. In severe cases with the following signs serum potassium >5 mmol/L, cardiac conduction abnormalities, arrhythmia, muscle twitching, etc, IV calcium chlorate or gluconate plus IV 10% dextrose with rapid-acting insulin is administered first while waiting for dialysis. Hyperphosphatemia is treated with phosphate intake restriction and elimination from IV solutions, avoidance of bicarbonates, and use of oral non-calcium phosphate binder. In severe cases renal replacement therapy may be suggested. Serum calcium levels get adjusted as the phosphate levels normalize.

139:
Answer: C.   Decrease in tumor size

Explanation: Delirium is common in terminally ill patients. It is characterized by rapidly emerging disturbance of consciousness and a change in cognition with fluctuating symptoms and evidence of organic etiology. Usually, terminally ill patients require sedation for delirium at that stage. Delirium in terminally ill patients may be due to the use of certain drugs like opioids, cessation of certain drugs like benzodiazepines, alcohol withdrawal symptoms, metabolic imbalance like hypercalcemia, renal failure, a primary tumor affecting the brain, metastasis of tumor in the brain. Successful treatment of tumors with a decrease in size and regeneration of normal cells will result in improvement of delirium and not worsening. Treatment of delirium is important as it may cause disturbance to those surrounding the person. Management includes both pharmacological and non-pharmacological measures. Delirium in the last few days of life is usually ongoing and irreversible, and in 20% of terminally ill patients sedation is the only treatment.

140:
Answer: B.   Decreased blood sugar levels

Explanation: Corticosteroids are drugs that help reduce inflammation in the body and also suppress the immune system. They are used to treat various diseases like asthma, severe allergy, weight gain, increased blood sugar levels, and osteoporosis (bone thinning). Corticosteroid alters the body's metabolism and prednisolone is known to cause the deposition of fat in the base or back of the neck and around the abdomen, leading to a moon face appearance with the face being more round. Alterations in electrolytes balance cause fluid retention and may increase blood pressure also. Long term steroid use commonly affects glucose metabolism and thus causes increased blood sugar levels. GI problems and increased infection risks are other common effects of steroid use. Steroid withdrawal may also be seen and hence tapering of steroids to when off is important.

141:
Answer: D.   Increased alertness

Explanation: Increased intracranial pressure can occur due to various reasons like brain tours, hemorrhage, and viral encephalitis. Increased ICP causes a decrease in cerebral perfusion which can lead to ischemia and cell death. Early signs and symptoms include changes in mental status like irritability, restlessness, and increased drowsiness. Other symptoms like decreased motor function and control, increased respiratory effort, nausea and vomiting, and seizures are also seen. Late signs and symptoms that are seen when the condition worsens include decreased respiratory and pulse rates, Cheyne-stokes respiration, lowered level of consciousness, and increased blood pressure and temperature. Diagnosis includes checking blood pressure, pupil dilation, spinal tap, and Cushing's triad.

142:
Answer: D.   By showing the daughter about the simple procedures such as mouth care

Explanation: When a patient is near death, the nurse's role is to support and guide the daughter in helping her mother. This includes simple procedures such as mouth care to make the patient more comfortable.

143:
Answer: B. PTH-related proteins that are osteoclastic released by tumor

Explanation: Hypercalcaemia is seen in 10-30% of cancer patients. Hypercalcemia is associated with increased osteoclastic bone resolution which can happen with or without bone metastases. It is mainly due to the release of parathyroid hormone-related protein from the tumor, which activates PTH receptors and thus leads to osteoclastic bone resorption and renal tubular resorption of calcium. Clinical features include dehydration, polyuria, polydipsia, nausea, vomiting, constipation, anorexia or neurologic Symptoms like fatigue, delirium, etc. Severe cases present with seizures, coma, or cardiovascular collapse. Normally treatment includes iv bisphosphonates and hydration with saline

144:
Answer: A.   Fluid retention

Explanation: Dexamethasone is typically given to patients prior to docetaxel in order to prevent fluid retention. Fluid retention can occur as a side effect of docetaxel and can lead to difficulty in breathing, chest pain, and an increased risk of heart attack or stroke. By giving dexamethasone ahead of time, the nurse can help to reduce the risk of these side effects.

145:
Answer: B.   To teach about a safe home environment
Explanation: In grade 3 peripheral neuropathy, the primary nursing intervention would be to teach about a safe home environment. This includes helping the patient to identify potential hazards in their home and teaching them how to safely navigate around these hazards. Other interventions may also be necessary depending on the individual patient's needs.

146:
Answer: C.   Autonomy
Explanation: Advanced directives are based on the principle of autonomy, which means that individuals have the right to make decisions about their own health care. Advanced directives allow individuals to specify what type of medical treatment they would want or not want if they are no longer able to make decisions for themselves.

147:
Answer: A.   Body's sense of positioning
Explanation: Romberg's test is a test used to examine the neurological function related to the body's sense of position (proprioception), i.e. balance without using vestibular function and vision. The patient is asked to stand and close his/her eyes, and if there is an increased loss of balance (more than a slight sway) then it is said to indicate a positive Romberg test. Positive Romberg signs suggest ataxia is due to loss of proprioception and a negative rompers test suggests ataxia if present is cerebellar. In cancer patients, the disease progression or the treatment may affect the patient's balance resulting in a positive Romberg's test. Hence healthcare workers must be aware of how to assess such patients and provide the treatment needed.

148:
Answer: C. Prostate-specific antigens

Explanation: A prostate-specific antigen (PSA) is a protein produced by the prostate gland. A high level of PSA in the blood may be a sign of prostate cancer.

149:
Answer: A. Acute lymphoblastic leukemia

Explanation: An allogeneic stem cell transplant is a treatment option for patients with acute lymphoblastic leukemia (ALL), a cancer of white blood cells. The transplant procedure involves receiving healthy stem cells from a donor to replace the patient's own destroyed or unhealthy stem cells. The donated stem cells create new, healthy blood cells, which can help to fight leukemia and improve the patient's prognosis.

150:
Answer: D. Ifosfamide

Explanation: Conditioning regimens prior to bone marrow transplant include monoclonal antibodies, chemotherapy, and radiation which prevent the recipient's body from rejecting the transplant, help kill cancer cells, and creates space for new blood cells to grow. Hemorrhagic cystitis is an earlier risk for those receiving iv cyclophosphamide compared to the oral route of administration. The urinary metabolite of cyclophosphamide, acrolein, is believed to be responsible for hemorrhagic cystitis. Mesna is given preventively to reduce the risk of hemorrhagic cystitis (HC) as it acts by altering the breakdown products of cyclophosphamide that affect the bladder. Alum is successfully used as an intravesical agent to treat HC. Sodium hyaluronate is a glycosaminoglycan present on the urinary bladder lining as a protective layer and various studies report its successful use to treat HC.

151:
Answer: A. Transfusion of platelets

Explanation: Cancer-related DIC presents in three forms- procoagulant, hyper fibrinolytic and subclinical. There is no single treatment option for DIC and it is altered according to the patient. While usual treatment is related to the cause of DIC, in this patient metastatic cancer is difficult to treat immediately and hence symptomatic and supportive care is the main focus along with continued normal treatment of cancer. Due to the platelet count being below 50,000/mcL is it advised to first provide a transfusion of platelets to the patient and get the level to between 30,000-50,000 at least. Administration of blood components like Plasma and/or factor transfusion is also given to keep PT and fibrinogen levels at a check of <3 and >5g/L respectively. Antifibrinolytic therapy is advised in specific cases like this where fibrinolytic activity is more, to reduce the FDP levels in this patient. Tranexamic acid is usually avoided as it has severe effects if not administered correctly and hence is never given alone and only when essential. Low molecular weight heparin is considered in cases where bleeding is not severe and it helps slow the coagulation process but in cases of brain metastasis, it must be used with caution due to the risk of intracranial hemorrhage.

152:
Answer: A.   **Anxiety**
Explanation: Anxiety is commonly associated with cancer patients, and it can range from mild to severe. A cancer diagnosis triggers feelings of fear for life, fear of treatments, or its side effects. This anxiety appears as reactive and repetitive behaviors like questioning diagnosis accuracy and disbelief. It is important for staff treating cancer patients to be aware of such signs and symptoms and support the patient through the process.

153:
Answer: D.   **Exercise**

Explanation: Constipation is a common side effect of cancer and its treatment. It is seen in over 60% of cancer patients. Constipation can be due to various reasons in cancer patients like tumor location, bacterial overgrowth, decreased activity, fatigue, drug induced due to opioids, anticholinergics, etc. Management of cancer-related constipation includes both nondrug and pharmacological management. Non-Drug management includes a higher fiber diet, exercise,and abdominal massage. However exercise is not commonly suggested due to the other stress of cancer. Even high fiber diets are advised in very few cases of low to moderate constipation cases. Pharmacological management includes the use of bulking agents, stool softeners like docusate, stimulants like bisacodyl, senna and enema; osmotic agents like magnesium citrate; lactulose, etc. These medications have to be used with caution for their side effects like bloating, gas, etc.

154:
Answer: B.   Methylphenidate
Explanation: It is likely that Cherry is experiencing fatigue due to medication side effects. The nurse would likely predict that methylphenidate would be the best stimulant to help alleviate Cherry's exhausted state.

155:
Answer: B.   Endoscopy
Explanation: Esophageal cancer is usually found due to the signs and symptoms presented by the patient. Various tests like barium swallow study, and CT scan are used to diagnose it. Endoscopy is an important test to diagnose esophageal cancer which includes upper endoscopy that may be accompanied by tissue biopsy and endoscopic ultrasound. While the early disease may not show any symptoms, the common ones experienced include difficulty in swallowing, unintentional weight loss, chest pain or burning, cough, and indigestion.

156:
Answer: C.   Altering patient position, steroids, radiation therapy, surgery

Explanation: Spinal cord compression is seen in 5-10 % of cancer patients and is most commonly seen in cancers of the breast, lung and prostate. It can occur due to a local increase in the size of cancer compressing the spinal cord or metastatic tumor spreading to the spinal cord. Signs and symptoms include worsening neck and back pain, motor weakness, numbness in arms and/or legs, and bladder issues. Treatments immediately first include altering the patient's position to lie straight on the back and administration of steroids to decrease swelling, then radiation therapy is commonly the treatment choice for radiosensitive tumors. Surgery may be used with or instead of radiation therapy for tumors with specific indications like an unknown primary tumor, the tumor is not responsive to radiation therapy and rapidly progressing neurological symptoms.

157:
Answer: B.   Increase use of sedative medication prior to meals

Explanation: Those patients who have dysphagia are at risk for aspiration which can lead to pneumonia and other issues. Hence various precautions need to be taken in such patients to ensure no aspiration occurs during eating or drinking. Patients with this risk include those who had a stroke, esophageal cancer or muscular dystrophies. The measures taken to prevent aspirations include - postural changes that allow better swallowing, upright /90 degree position while eating and 30 minutes after food intake, adjusting the viscosity of food to allow better intake which includes the use of thickening agents, avoiding rushed or forced feedings, reducing the use of drugs like sedatives which impair swallowing and cough reflexes, alternate solids and liquids consumption, providing 30 minutes rest prior to eating which allows the patient to swallow better. Signs of aspiration that need to be looked out for include sudden respiratory symptoms like severe coughing, change in voice after eating, pocketing of food on one side.

158:
Answer: D.   Apply lotion with Dimethicone

Explanation: Robin reports yellow, crusty papules and itching on her shoulder. This could be a sign of an allergic reaction to the therapy and she should apply a topical lotion with Dimethicone.

159:

Answer: D. **Decreased heart rate**

Explanation: Cardiac tamponade is a medical condition caused due to increased accumulation of pericardial pressure which leads to impaired cardiac filling and hemodynamic compromise. It can occur due to bacterial infection, cancer, autoimmune disease, or radiation to the chest area. While in subacute cardiac tamponade there may be no symptoms. The symptoms eventually appear and they are severe and sudden in acute cardiac tamponade like chest pain, shortness of breathing, fast breathing, enlargement of neck veins, decreased blood pressure, increased heart rate, light headedness. Diagnosis includes ECG, echocardiogram, CT or MRI. Blood tests may also be required to identify infections, autoimmune disease, etc. Immediate treatment usually includes pericardiocentesis in emergency cases and otherwise, radiation or surgery is planned to remove the extra pericardial fluids . Other measures include treating the cause, regular monitoring with ECGs, etc.

160:

Answer: A. **No gloves are needed while handling them**

Explanation: Individuals who prepare or administer hazardous drugs like some of those used for cancer treatment, some antivirals, etc must take special care. Exposure to such drugs may lead to carcinogenesis, teratogenesis, infertility, or genotoxicity. The health risk depends on the amount of exposure, duration and drug type. Adverse skin reactions are a common effect leading to contact dermatitis with symptoms of redness, rash, etc. Hence use of gloves and other protective equipment during its preparation, administration and disposal is essential. Various engineering precautions including proper ventilation systems will help prevent accidental exposure to these hazardous drugs. Cisplatin, etoposide, and Fluorouracil are examples of such hazardous drugs.

161:

Answer: B. **Discussing about the Palliative sedation initiation with the team.**

Explanation: The nurse's next plan of action would be to discuss palliative sedation with the team. Palliative sedation is a type of sedation that is used to reduce pain and discomfort in patients with terminal illnesses. The goal of palliative sedation is to make the patient as comfortable as possible.

162:
Answer: B. **A gene that has the ability to become a transformer gene by transforming a normal cell into the cancer cell**
Explanation: Proto-oncogenes are genes that have the ability to become tumor-promoting or oncogenes by transforming a normal cell into a cancer cell. They are normal genes that can be mutated or activated to promote tumor growth. Oncogenes are a type of proto-oncogene.

163:
Answer: D. **As long as the patient wishes to consume food and water.**
Explanation: A hospice patient nearing death should be given food and water till the patient wishes to consume food and water. This is based on the principle of autonomy, which is the right of individuals to self-determination. Patients should be allowed to make their own decisions about their care, including whether or not they want to eat and drink. If the patient has lost the ability to make decisions for themselves, then their power of attorney or another legal representative should make decisions on their behalf.

164:
Answer: B. **Superior Vena Cava Syndrome (SVCS)**
Explanation: Superior Vena Cava Syndrome (SVCS) is a condition that is caused by obstruction of the superior vena cava (SVC), which is the large vein that carries blood from the upper body to the heart. When the SVC is blocked, blood can back up into the veins in the head and neck, causing swelling and other symptoms. SVCS can be a sign of advanced lung cancer, and it can also occur with other types of cancer that spread to the chest. Symptoms of SVCS include swelling in the face, neck, arms, and hands; distended veins in the head, neck, and chest; disturbed vision; headache; and disorientation. If you suspect that someone you know has SVCS due to lung cancer, seek medical attention right away.

165:
Answer: A.   **Preserving the bladder function**

Explanation: The main goal in treating muscle-invasive bladder cancer is to preserve bladder function. This can be done by surgically removing cancer while preserving as much of the bladder as possible. If cancer cannot be removed surgically, radiation therapy may be used to help shrink the tumor and preserve the bladder.

166:
Answer: C.   **Methotrexate**

Explanation: Chemotherapeutic drugs while used to treat cancer have various side effects also. Out of these effects on the fertility of the patient is one. In males, certain drugs may lead to azoospermia/oligospermia and in females, it may lead to ovarian failure. The side effects may be temporary or permanent and are also sometimes dose-dependent. Alkylating agents like busulfan, ifosfamide, cyclophosphamide, cisplatin, and procarbazine are the most gonadotoxic drugs and cause direct destruction to the oocytes and follicular depletion. Methotrexate treatment even long term is very rarely linked to fertility issues and is seen mostly when other drugs are also being used in the treatment plan.

167:
Answer: C.   **A dull, grey stoma**

Explanation: Robert notices that the skin around his colostomy is dull and grey. This is likely due to the accumulation of drainage and secretions around the stoma.

168:
Answer: B.   **Pharmacological management is a must**

Explanation: Dyspnea is basically shortness or difficulty in breathing. It is a common symptom in cancer patients with or without lung involvement. The cause of dyspnea in cancer patients can be due to direct cancer involvement of lungs, indirectly related to cancer effects like anemia, and cachexia. Management includes general and pharmacological management. General measures include altering bed positions, discontinuing parenteral fluids, and bedside relaxation techniques. Pharmacological management first includes the use of opioids either oral or parenteral, anxiolytics like lorazepam, anticholinergics like scopolamine and also treatment with oxygen for hypoxia.

169:
Answer: C.   Lower back pain, loss of leg function and bladder control
Explanation: Lumbar- sacral spinal cord compression can be due to various reasons like tumors or trauma. Spinal compression in this area affects the middle and lower body, not the upper body. Signs and symptoms include lower back pain, paralysis or decreased sensation of legs, loss of bladder and bowel control (incontinence), foot drop. Lumbar compression is associated with cauda equina syndrome.

170:
Answer: A.   Prevents accumulation of lymph in soft tissue
Explanation: Multi-layered lymphoedema bandaging (MLLB) is used as a treatment method for lymphedema. The main goal of using a compression garment is to prevent lymph build-up in soft tissues and allow it to drain. This compression treatment involved outing even and firm pressure on the tissues involved. This pressure helps the trapped lymph fluid to flow through the vessels and reduce swelling.

171:
Answer: D.   Cancer prevention is more

Explanation: Poverty increases the risk of cancer mortality rates. Those with lower socioeconomic status are likely to have a higher incidence of cancer and lower survival rates. Irrespective of the cancer site, the survival rates are lower among the poor. Disparity with regard to factors that affect cancer like nutrition, obesity, substance abuse, etc becomes more obvious. Lack of a proper diet increases the risk for cancer. Regular screening for cancer is also lesser among the poor and especially the uneducated. Daily life stresses increase among the poor and hence they have less time to focus on the prevention of cancer which includes healthy lifestyles, genetic mapping, etc. lower socioeconomic status individuals are at a higher risk of being diagnosed with advanced-stage cancers due to lack of screening and delayed healthcare.

172:
Answer: D.   Changing prescribed medicine and its dosage
Explanation: It is important that family members or those who will be with the patient at home be aware of the appropriate care to be given to the cancer patient. It is the responsibility of the oncology nurse to train the family member/house member on how to take care of the patient. This includes management of symptoms of cancer and treatment side effects, administration of correct prescribed drugs according to doctors' instructions, management of medical emergencies, emotional support, management and use of iv cannula, what to do in case of fever, emergency numbers to be contacted. Making the home physically accessible and safe for the patient is also important which may include handrails, non-slip surfaces,andb wheelchair access.

173:
Answer: D.   Cancer cells migrate to the neighboring locations and tissues
Explanation: Cancer cells are distinctly different from other cells in a few ways. First, cancer cells typically have the ability to migrate to neighboring locations and tissues. They can also invade and damage other healthy tissues. Additionally, cancer cells often lack the normal controls that keep cell growth in check, which can lead to unchecked tumor growth. Finally, cancer cells often produce abnormal amounts of proteins that promote tumor growth and survival.

174:
Answer: D. **The patient can be advised to return to normal activities immediately after treatment**

Explanation: Testicular cancer and its treatment have various effects on the patient and proper explanation and management of these effects is a vital part of a nurse's care plan. Orchiectomy may involve the removal of one or both testicles and requires hospital admission for a few days post procedure and pain management. Testicular self examination must be taught to the patient to help in the early diagnosis of any new or recurrent tumor. Removal of one or both testicles may affect the patient's testosterone levels and hormone therapy may be needed. Sexual dysfunction may also be experienced by the patient and sperm collection prior to surgery must be discussed.

175:
Answer: A. **It needs to be flushed before and after every use**

Explanation: An Implantable venous access device is useful to have long-term and repeated access to the bloodstream of the patient for antibiotics, nutrition, etc. It can be left in place for years together and removed when not needed anymore. It consists of a catheter and a port which are implanted under the skin with access usually to a large vein. When the device needs to be used then a special small, right angled needle is inserted into the port. Flushing of the port must be done before and after every use, and once a month if not used. Implantable venous access device placement is usually an outpatient procedure, done under radiological guidance to ensure the correct position of device.

176:
Answer:D. **Needs to be replaced every two weeks**

Explanation: A peripherally inserted central catheter (PICC) is a tube that is inserted into a vein above the elbow (rarely leg) and is then guided to the central vein for intravenous access. It allows administration of various medications, nutrition, etc and also drawing of blood when needed to be done regularly. It can stay in place for weeks or a couple of months. It'll prevent vein injury due to multiple needle pricks and also prevents irritation of small veins due to iv medications. It can be used in hospital and home setups and must be regularly flushed.

177:
Answer: A.   Escitalopram

Explanation: Generalised anxiety for patients in palliative care is quite common due to the uncertainty of living with an illness and the possibility of death. It includes feelings of worry, restlessness, loneliness, fear of future or death, or disturbed sleep. Various studies have proven that untreated and persistent anxiety worsens the condition of the patient. Treatment for anxiety in cancer patients in palliative care may include psychotherapy, medications, and lifestyle modifications. Serotonin reuptake inhibitors (SSRI) like escitalopram and citalopram, are the first-line medications used to treat general anxiety disorders. Other medications like benzodiazepines may also be used.

178:
Answer: A.   **Discuss the importance of delaying conception, fetal damage due to treatment, surrogacy, embryo preservation, etc.**

Explanation: Cancer and its treatment affect patients' reproductive and sexual health in multiple ways like infertility, loss of sexual desire, etc. Possible pregnancy during cancer is not encouraged and delaying pregnancy up to 1 year after cancer treatment is suggested. This helps any damaged eggs to leave the body and also the chance of recurrence of cancer is more likely during this period. Chemotherapy and radiotherapy are known to have teratogenic effects on the fetus and thus may lead to fetal abnormalities. Cancer treatment is known to lower the patient's immunity thus putting them at increased risk for STIs also, thus proper protection is important. Alternative options including IVF, surrogacy, adoption, sperm preservation, etc must be discussed with patients clearly to ensure they are aware of the choices in case of fertility issues post-treatment.

179:
Answer: A. (HUS) SIADH syndrome

Explanation: Small cell lung cancer (SCLC) is a particularly aggressive form of lung cancer. Early signs and symptoms can be subtle and nonspecific, including weight gain, headaches, and excessive thirst. SCLC often spreads quickly to other parts of the body, so it's important to seek medical attention if you experience any of these symptoms.

180:
Answer: D.   increased fibrin degradation products

Explanation: Disseminated intravascular coagulation is a syndrome characterized by intravascular coagulation due to various reasons and not at any specific location. Whatever the cause, it can lead to microvascular damage and in severe cases also lead to organ dysfunction. There is the activation of coagulation pathways, excess intravascular fibrin formation, and excessive thrombin generation with widespread microvascular thrombosis which can lead to ischemia and consumption of platelets and coagulation factors. There is an exhaustion of coagulation proteases, decreased clotting factors as they are used up, a low platelet count which leads to diffuse bleeding, elevated D-dimer concentration, decreased fibrinogen concentration and increased fibrin degradation products, and prolongation of clotting times such as prothrombin time (PT). Treatment includes treatment of underlying cause and transfusion and anticoagulant therapy.

181:
Answer: C. BRCA1
Explanation: Biologic response modifiers (BRM) are substances that modify the immune system response which are naturally produced in the body or can be made in the lab. They help in treating various autoimmune diseases by targeting the disease mechanism. They also help treat certain cancers like non-hodgkin's lymphoma. Examples of these are interferons, interleukins, monoclonal antibodies, TNF inhibitors, rituximab, infliximab, and colony stimulating factors. Some of the side effects include nausea, vomiting, diarrhea, loss of appetite, fever, skin rash, increased bleeding tendency, etc. BRCA1 Is a gene whose mutation is commonly associated with a high risk of breast cancer.

182:
Answer: D.   African Americans

Explanation: Although cancer occurs to people from any race or ethnicity, statistically it has been proven that mortality due to cancer has a higher incidence among African-Americans. Lung, prostate and colorectal cancer were the main types of cancers that caused mortality in African-Americans compared to other ethnicities. Risk factors among this ethnicity mainly include obesity and smoking. Asian and pacific islanders had the least cancer mortality rates among the various ethnicities studied. While African-Americans have the highest mortality due to cancer and the least survival rate.

183:
Answer: D.   By asking a question without any hesitation in order to acquire more knowledge

Explanation: When helping a patient in doing a life review, the ideal approach is to ask questions without any hesitation in order to acquire more knowledge. It is crucial to understand the patient's perspective and feelings about their life in order to provide support and advice. If the patient is uncomfortable speaking about certain aspects of their life, it is important to be respectful and understanding. By being open and compassionate, the therapist can create a safe and supportive environment for the patient to explore their life experiences.

184:
Answer: C.   Scientific evidence

Explanation: Evidence based practice basically means practice done based on the evidence available related to it which may be from scientific research, statistics, professional experience, etc. It may not be peer-reviewed. The scientific evidence is derived from well-designed clinical trials. The personal choice of the doctor is not included as it may be biased and does not have any clear basis for being chosen. It is important that the doctor be aware of all new data related to the specific practice and take it into account while making decisions. Medically supported data is given the highest importance for being the deciding factor behind doctors' advice/decisions.

185:
Answer: B.   Cleaning hazardous drug spill

Explanation: The National Institute for Occupational Safety and Health (NIOSH) recommends wearing a respirator when cleaning up hazardous spills. This is because there is a risk of inhaling the chemicals or particles in the air. A respirator can protect your lungs from these hazards.

186:
Answer: D.   **Prostate cancer**

Explanation: While radiotherapy is used to treat cancer it is also sadly known to put the patient at risk for secondary radiation-induced malignancies. The risk of developing secondary malignancies is currently about 17-19% and the risk increases based on the type of lifestyle genetics, treatment modality etc. Radiotherapy puts the person at higher risk for certain types of secondary malignancies. Bone and soft tissue sarcomas for example angiosarcoma are the most common radiation-induced secondary malignancies. Breast cancer is also a possible common sequela of chest radiation, including certain leukemias. Cancers of the brain, prostate, etc are least likely to occur due to chest radiation.

187:
Answer: A.   **Check blood potassium, calcium, and magnesium levels are normal**

Explanation: Arsenic trioxide is currently approved for the treatment of APL. Cardiac effects of arsenic due to acute or chronic poisoning are well documented. Cardiovascular toxicity and fatal arrhythmias may occur as a side effects. Proper regular cardiac monitoring during treatment with arsenic is hence vital so early signs of cardiac toxicity can be detected, otherwise, the outcome may be fatal. This involves monitoring any changes in the QTc interval which is affected by hypocalcemia, hypomagnesemia and hypokalaemia. Hence monitoring of blood levels of potassium, magnesium and calcium must be done regularly.

188:
Answer: D.   **Etoposide**

Explanation: Carcinogenic medications are medications that can cause cancer. One such carcinogenic medication is etoposide. Etoposide is a chemotherapy drug that is used to treat different types of cancer, including leukemia, lung cancer, and testicular cancer. It works by killing cancer cells. However, it can also cause some serious side effects, including hair loss, nausea, and vomiting.

189:
Answer: A.   Increased clarity about their life choices
Explanation: Loss of personal control is basically the lack of the ability to provide conscious limitation of impulses and behavior as a result of overwhelming emotion. Patients diagnosed with cancer or other chronic illness may feel extremely overwhelmed and the disease itself may reduce the patient's personal control. The patient has no clarity about his life and choices, hence it leads to the person feeling extremely agitated and angry due to uncertainty. The patient may suddenly start weeping or say he is unable to do anything and is in a state of shock-like. There is increased frustration due to the inability to perform everyday tasks and an increased dependency on others. Patients will show signs of rebellious nature which include refusing treatment, fighting with doctors, etc. Whether this loss of personal control has serious effects on the safety of the patient and those around him/her must also be assessed carefully and all the necessary therapeutic measures must be undertaken. Patients with a history of trauma like child abuse may react to various triggers during the diagnosis and treatment, and hence such issues must be identified and handled wisely.

190:
Answer: C.   Haloperidol
Explanation: Yes, there is a medication that can treat delirium in patients who are dying. Haloperidol is a drug that is used to treat psychosis, and it has been shown to be effective in treating delirium in terminal patients.

191:
Answer: B.   Stage II

Explanation: Staging helps in understanding the spread of cancer in the patient's body and deciding a treatment plan or modification of the treatment plan as needed. Adult NHL is staged according to Lugano classification based on the Ann Arbor system. In Stage II either of the following is seen-
(1) The lymphoma is in 2 or more groups of lymph nodes on the same side of (above or below) the diaphragm (the thin band of muscle that separates the chest and abdomen) or (2) The lymphoma is in a group of lymph node(s) and in one area of a nearby organ (IIE) and it may also affect other groups of lymph nodes on the same side of the diaphragm. NHL in children is classified with the St. Jude system which also has 4 stages.

192:
Answer: D. Nurses must have knowledge about sexual health care and show a willingness to ask patients about it.
Explanation: Sexual health care is an important aspect of cancer and its treatment. It is important for oncology nurses to have the sexual knowledge necessary to understand the biological, psychological, and social aspects of sexual issues his/her patient may face. Cancer can affect sexual health in various ways including infertility, loss of sexual drive, etc. Various studies have shown that nurses lack the knowledge and/or are hesitant to bring up this topic and don't include it in patient care. Instead of burdening the patient to be the one to bring up any sexual issue, it is important the nurses bring up this topic in a respectable and sensitive manner. Continuing education and training related to sexual health care of cancer patients must be undertaken by nurses to ensure holistic care is offered to the patients.

193:
Answer: A.   An IgE mediated allergic reaction

Explanation: Anaphylaxis is a serious allergic reaction that starts rapidly and resents with various symptoms like itchy skin, vomiting, dizziness, shortness of breath, low BP, etc and may ultimately lead to death. IgE antibodies play an important role in anaphylaxis which occurs upon exposure to an allergen the person is previously sensitized to, and it acts on basophils and mast cells which trigger the release of histamine, leukotriene, and other mediators. It usually occurs 15-20 minutes after exposure to the allergen and late reactions may occur 4-8 hours later. Treatment includes administration of adrenaline, antihistamines, beta-receptor- agonists for bronchoconstriction, IV fluids, and intubation if needed.

194:
Answer: B. A 25-year-old patient receiving chemotherapy and radiation for Hodgkin lymphoma

Explanation: Radiation therapy can cause bone marrow depression, which is a decrease in the number of blood cells produced by the bone marrow. This can lead to anemia, neutropenia, and thrombocytopenia. Patients who are younger are at higher risk of bone marrow depression after radiation therapy than older patients.

195:
Answer: D. Programmed cell death

Explanation: Cancer development is a complex process but is simply explained by the occurrence of three stages in cell transformation which include initiation, promotion, and progression. Exposure to various carcinogens may trigger mutations in normal cells (initiation), then various internal and external promoters trigger the division (promotion) of these mutated cells uncontrollably due to loss of apoptosis (programmed cell death). During progression, there is further division and mutations of the cancer cells.

196:
Answer: A. Cytogenetic Analysis

Explanation: Cytogenetic analysis involves analyses of cells obtained from various tissues of the body to check for chromosomal abnormalities which can be indicative of diseases. Bone marrow biopsy involves the removal of the soft tissue in the center of most large bones called bone marrow and is done using a needle. Various malignant conditions can be checked for by cytogenetic analysis of the bone marrow like leukemia and the results will further help in treatment planning.

197:
Answer: B.   Professional performance
Explanation: The nurse must exhibit behavioral approval for professional performance in order to take the oncology certified nurse examination. This means that they must follow the practice standards set by the Oncology Nursing Society. This includes things like providing competent, safe care to patients, respecting patient autonomy, and collaborating with other health care professionals.

198:
Answer: C.   The number of people who have specific cancer divided by the population at risk
Explanation: Cancer incidence basically refers to the number of people who got a specific type of cancer divided by the number of people at risk usually per year. It is usually written as the number of cancer cases per 100,000 people in the general population. Incidence can vary due to various factors like age, race, genetics, or gender. With an increase in age, there is an increased incidence of cancer and men are more likely to get cancer. Cancer prevalence refers to the number of people in the population who have a cancer diagnosis- including both new and existing patients.

199:
Answer: D.   NIOSH List of Antineoplastic and Other Hazardous Drugs in Healthcare Setting

Explanation: The NIOSH List of Antineoplastic and Other Hazardous Drug in Healthcare Setting is a reference that can aid the nurse in determining the characteristics and safe handling measures of a potentially hazardous medicine. The list includes information on specific drugs such as their chemical name, common trade name, and proposed labeling. It also includes information on recommended safe handling measures for nurses, such as wearing gloves and using personal protective equipment.

200:
Answer: D.   Filtered

Explanation: Communication between cancer patients and healthcare workers is very important. It has huge effects on the patient's treatment, compliance, and beliefs. It is important to maintain smooth communication and ensure it is mainly client-focused as long as the client is physically and mentally sound. Filtered communication is basically when the doctor and patient alone, directly talk about the patient's diagnosis, and then the patient conveys the information he/she wishes to his family members. This allows the patient to be in control of the information shared with his/her significant others.

201:
Answer: C.   Agranulocytosis

Explanation: Sepsis is a life-threatening condition that involves the dramatic response of the immune system to an infection, usually bacterial, where the patient's own tissue is damaged and organs do not function properly. Signs and symptoms include high fever, breathing difficulty, confusion, increased heart rate. There are many risk factors for sepsis but the most important in a cancer patient undergoing chemotherapy is agranulocytosis which occurs due to various cancer-drugs. While old age or very young age, comorbid conditions like diabetes, liver diseases, intravenous devices, and prolonged hospital stay are also important factors to consider, the unique factor in cancer patients undergoing treatment is agranulocytosis where the neutrophil levels are extremely low and the patient's ability to fight infection is very low. Treatment includes altering drug dosage, use of antibiotics and treatment of infection.

202:

Answer: B.   Delayed

Explanation: Chemotherapy-induced nausea is a common side-effect of chemotherapy. There are three types of chemotherapy-induced nausea: anticipatory, acute, and delayed. Delayed nausea is the most common type, and it can occur up to 24 hours after chemotherapy has been administered. Symptoms include nausea, vomiting, and an upset stomach. Treatment for delayed nausea usually includes antiemetics such as ondansetron or promethazine.

203:
Answer: A.   The nurse should apply some ice and administer dexrazoxane.

Explanation: The nurse should first apply some ice to the site to help control the swelling. They should then administer dexrazoxane, which is a drug that helps protect against the damaging effects of anthracyclines.

204:
Answer: D.   Inform the blood transfusion center about the patient's use of this drug

Explanation: Daratumumab binds to CD38 and may mask the antibodies detection which will interfere with compatibility testing done prior to blood transfusion and result in false positive. Coombs test up to 6 months after treatment. This will in turn lead to a delay in the transfusion process. Hence to prevent this it's advised to test for blood compatibility prior to administration of Daratumumab or to use a DTT-treated reagent during the Coombs test if Daratumumab is already administered.

205:
Answer: B.   Bone metastases and hypercalcemia

Explanation: The current patient's condition is indicative of recurrent breast cancer with osteolytic metastasis related to hypercalcemia. While hypercalcemia due to malignancy can be due to a varied number of reasons, bone metastases are most common in breast cancer. The bone scan may show osteolytic lesions indicative of this. Hormone receptor-negative breast cancer is more prone to early recurrence i.e. within five years of treatment. Proper assessment of patients for recurrence of cancer, bone lesions, serum calcium and phosphate levels must all be assessed and treatment is done accordingly.

206:
Answer: B.   T3N2M1
Explanation: In TNM staging, T refers to the degree of invasion, N refers to the nodal involvement and M refers to distant metastasis. T1 means the tumor has grown into layers below mucosa like lamina propria or muscularis mucosa or submucosa. T2 means the tumor has grown into muscularis propria. T3 means subserosa layer is affected. T4a is when the stomach wall is affected but not nearby organs and T4b is when the stomach wall and nearby organs or structures are affected. N1 is where 1-2 nearby lymph nodes are involved. N2 is where 3-6 nearby lymph nodes are involved. N3a is when 7-15 nearby lymph nodes are affected and N3b is when 16 or more nearby lymph nodes are affected. M1 Is the presence of distant metastasis. Thus a staging of T3N2M1 will have a poor prognosis.

207:
Answer: A.   Assess for possible anastomotic leak
Explanation: Anastomotic leakage is one of the most serious complications after gastric and esophageal surgery. Various reasons including ischemia of conduit and surgical technique contribute to this which becomes apparent on the 5-8th postoperative day with signs of fever, pain, lab reports showing increased creatinine, etc. Due to the associated risk of mortality and complications, a routine water-soluble contrast swallow is done post-operatively, as early as possible, to help diagnose and treat it at the earliest.

208:
Answer: B.   Is intended to relieve refractory status in dying patients

Explanation: Terminal or Palliative sedation is basically carried out to relieve refractory symptoms in dying/terminally ill patients. The most common refractory symptoms for palliative sedation are delirium, intractable pain, and shortness of breath, but there is no clear definition of refractory symptoms. It is usually carried out when traditional therapies are not effective anymore or their doses needed have more adverse effects. Well-documented goals of care must be clearly discussed with the patient and his/her family members. The main aim is not to sedate the patient but to alleviate the symptoms. The dose of medications used must be as needed to provide specific clinical effects. An example of medications used is benzodiazepines, opiates, and antipsychotics to alleviate patients' respiratory distress, agitation, and anxiety and cause sedation.

209:
Answer: B.   Apoptosis
Explanation: The hallmarks of cancer were originally six, and now there are eight biological capabilities of cancer cells along with two enabling capabilities. The main characteristics of cancer cells are - (1) self-sufficiency in growth signals; (2) insensitivity to anti-growth hormones; (3) no apoptosis; (4) limitless replication ; (5) sustained angiogenesis ; (6) tissue invasion and metastasis ; (7) deregulated metabolism; (8) evading the immune system. Enabling characteristics which lead to cancer cell development include genome instability and inflammation.

210:
Answer: C.   Blood reports show normal RBC and calcium levels

Explanation: Multiple myeloma is a cancer that affects plasma cells which are a type of white blood cells and is more common in males, older age and blacks. These abnormal cells crowd out regular blood cells and thus lead to anemia and also trigger osteoclastic activity which leads to bone degradation and hypercalcemia in blood. Symptoms include bone pain, weakness, upset stomach, frequent infections, and severe thirst. Kidney problems may also be seen in multiple myeloma. Common treatment includes chemotherapy with drugs like cyclophosphamide, bendamustine, immunomodulatory drugs like thalidomide, lenalidomide, etc. Radiation therapy and immunotherapy may also be used to treat it. Stem cell transplant along with other treatment modalities is also strongly advised. Choice of treatment will depend on the stage of cancer.

211:

Answer: C. Radiation therapy

Explanation: Lungs are very sensitive to radiation and hence radiation therapy that affects these tissues may lead to radiation-related lung injury. Even chemotherapy may lead to pulmonary toxicity. The use of both of the above therapies to treat cancers like lung, breast or esophageal cancer leads to an increased risk of pulmonary toxicity. These risks are often related to the doses of treatment and hence lung toxicity acts as dose-limiting factor. Radiation-induced lung damage is often limited to the exposed areas and includes various side effects like pneumonia, fibrosis, and other respiratory disorders. The preexisting lung condition, dosage and duration of treatment, age, and steroid use affect the lung toxicity due to radiation/chemo--therapy. Various preventive measures are being studied which include mitigators, modifiers, and protectors, which may help prevent this lung toxicity like ACE (angiotensin-converting enzyme) inhibitors, Amifostine.

212:

Answer: D. The warn act

Explanation: Cancer survivors are protected according to various laws when it comes to their employment and rehabilitation. The ADA prohibits job discrimination by employers, employment agencies and labour unions against people who have or had cancer. The federal rehabilitation act was before the ADA and it prevents public and private employers that receive public funds from discriminating based on disability. The FMLA requires those with 50 or more employees to provide 12 weeks of unpaid, job-protected leave for family members who need time off to address their own or their family member's serious health illnesses. According to the Warn Act if there is an employment site shutdown or mass layoff, employees must be given 60 days' notice.

213:
Answer: C. 195/mm3
Explanation: Absolute Neutrophil Count (ANC) helps assess the body's ability to fight infections, especially bacterial infections. An ANC measures the number of neurophils in the blood. Neutrophils are a type of white blood cell that kills bacteria. The absolute neutrophil count is calculated by multiplying total neutrophils percentage (segmented and bands) and multiplying by the white blood cell count and dividing by In this case - (32+7=+39) x 500 ÷100 = 195/mm. A healthy person has an ANC between 1500 and 6000. A lesser value of ANC leads to neutropenia resulting in an increased risk of infection.

214:
Answer: B.   Addresses patient's concerns before starting the treatment
Explanation: The nurse's plan now is to address the patient's concerns before starting the treatment. This will help ensure that the patient understands the treatment and is comfortable with moving forward. If there are any remaining questions or concerns, the nurse can address those at that time as well.

215:
Answer: B. Infection at site and systemic

Explanation: Infection is the most common and also most preventable CVAD complication, which can be systemic or localized. When the infection spreads from the catheter into the bloodstream it leads to bacteremia. Various measures can be taken to prevent this which includes following proper hand hygiene while handling CVAD, proper disinfection methods followed, aseptic technique followed during infusion therapy administrations and all CVAD dressing changes; changing administration sets and addon devices at appropriate intervals; maintaining a closed infusion system; and removing CVADs when they're no longer necessary. Risk factors for infection related to CVAD include immunocompromised individuals, severe chronic illness, leukopenia, very young or very old age. Symptoms of infection include fever, chills, nausea, vomiting, backache. Treatment if the infection is suspected includes blood cultures, removal of catheter, and antibiotic administration as needed.

216:
Answer: B. Osteolytic bone metastases
Explanation: Hypercalcemia due to malignancy is common in the late stages of cancer. Calcium levels in the body are regulated by a variety of mechanisms including PTH, Vitamin-D, and calcitonin. PTHrP is produced by various cells normally including breast cells, and under normal conditions helps in calcium transport. Malignancies like breast cancer, squamous cell carcinoma, etc lead to hypercalcemia by increased PTHrP action which causes increased renal calcium absorption and increased osteoclastic activity. Multiple myeloma and breast cancer are the major malignancies that cause hypercalcemia by osteolytic metastasis which causes excessive release of calcium from the bones. Metastasis to the bone in breast cancer triggers growth factor β, which stimulates PTHrP to be produced by metastatic breast cancer cells and in multiple myeloma triggers various cytokines like RANKL that lead to hypercalcemia.

217:
Answer: A. Complementary and alternative medicine

Explanation: Complementary and alternative medicine (CAM) basically refers to medical practices and products that are not standard western medical care. Complementary medicine is used along with standard treatment and alternative treatment may be used instead of standard treatment. The five categories are - (1) mind-body therapy- meditation, tai chi, hypnosis, etc.; (2) biologically based practices- botanicals, special diets, etc; (3) manipulative and body based practices- chiropractic therapy, reflexology, etc; (4) biofield therapy- reiki, etc; (5) whole medical systems- ayurveda, homeopathy, etc. These practices may help cancer patients cope with side effects of standard treatments, comfort them, and may cure the disease.

218:
Answer: A.   Translation by the patient's spouse is not recommended
Explanation: Translation by the patient's spouse is not recommended because it can lead to inaccuracies and misunderstandings. Most hospitals have interpreters on staff who are qualified to translate medical information accurately.

219:
Answer: C.   By allowing the patient to express her feelings
Explanation: The nurse will most likely react to the patient with understanding and support. It is likely that the nurse will have some knowledge of lymphedema and what to expect for patients who have developed the condition. The nurse will offer comfort and assurance to the patient, letting her know that she is not alone in her struggle.

220:
Answer: C. Cell-Mediated
Explanation: Acquired immunity is of two types- cell-mediated or humoral. Cell-mediated immunity is that immunity that involves mature T- cells, macrophages and cytokines which are responsible for intracellular destruction of antigens including microbes, viruses, etc. It does not involve antibodies. Humoral immunity is an antibody-mediated response to antigens that are mainly driven by B-cells that produce antibodies.

221:
Answer: C.   A highly similar medication that has the same therapeutic and clinical effects.

Explanation: Biosimilar drugs are basically highly similar drugs that have minor structural or chemical differences from the original product and are made after the patent of the original product expires. They have the same clinical and therapeutic effects as the original drug. Biosimilars are basically modeled after the original biological drug, which was the first in the market, without being an identical copy of it but having similar efficacy.

222:
Answer: B.   Same goal of team members

Explanation: There is an increase in desire to have collaboration relationships between different healthcare workers and/or administrative workers. While it is ideal for there to be perfect understanding, decision making process, trust, respect, etc amongst the team members, there are many barriers to this. These barriers may be organizational like lack of knowledge or appreciation for other roles, legal issues of scope and liability, etc; or at team level like lack of commitment of team members, different goals of members, etc; or at the individual level like split loyalties, lack is trust in the collaboration, gender/class/race prejudices, legal liability for others decisions, etc. It is important to overcome such barriers by proper communication, learning about other professions, respect for others' skills and knowledge, being willing to share responsibilities.

223:
Answer: B. Ileal conduit

Explanation: urinary diversions after radical cystectomy can be divided into three categories- incontinent urinary diversions, continent cutaneous urinary diversions, and orthotopic ileal neobladders. Various complications are associated with urinary diversion which include early complications like urine leakage, UTI, etc and late complications like renal failure, urolithiasis, metabolic abnormalities. Ileal conduits are known to lead to decreased urinary excretion of calcium and also hyperoxaluria which may commonly lead to stone formation. While ileal conduits are the most common and simple diversions, they have commonly been associated with the asymptomatic presence of bacteria in urine and in the long term urinary tract infections are common. As it is an incontinent urinary diversion, the reflux of contents is more common and leads to complications.

224:
Answer: B.   Myelin sheath
Explanation: The cells that give rise to oligodendroglia tumors maintain myelin sheath. Myelin sheath is a layer of electrically insulating material that surrounds the axons of some nerve cells. It helps to speed up the conduction of nerve impulses. Oligodendroglia tumors are tumors that arise from oligodendrocytes, which are the cells that produce myelin sheath.

225:
Answer: A.   Writing the first and last name
Explanation: Cytarabine is a drug commonly used to treat cancer. It has various side effects that affect the bone, GI system and CNS. Neurotoxicity is a potential adverse effect that needs to be assessed prior to the administration of high doses of cytarabine. Cerebellar assessments include various components like checking for speech impairments, gait, consciousness levels, handwriting changes, romberg test, etc. Early recognition of neurological symptoms and timely intervention will help decrease the severity and possibility of long-term complications. Multiple factors that contribute to neurotoxicity due to cytarabine are age, dosage, frequency of drug administration, and renal disease.

226:

Answer: A. Preserving the sperm before initiating the treatment

Explanation: The nurse will make a recommendation for Robert to preserve his sperm before initiating the treatment. This will ensure that he is able to conceive children in the future.

227:

Answer: D. A patient with decreased sensory perception

Explanation: People who have decreased sensory perception are more prone to skin breakdown because they cannot feel when their skin is damaged. This can lead to the development of pressure ulcers.

228:

Answer: B. MRI

Explanation: The most common cancers diagnosed in pregnant women are breast cancer, haematological malignancies, gynaecological malignancies, GI, and thyroid cancer. While cancer imaging is done in pregnant women it is important that the risk to the mother and fetus be assessed properly. MRI and Ultrasound are the safest and most preferred diagnostic methods due to lack of any ionizing radiations. MRI has the advantage of being clinically accurate, useful in distant staging through the whole body. CT, nuclear imaging, bone scan, etc that have ionizing radiation are only used in cases where the maternal benefit outweighs the fetal risk and radiation to the fetus is tried to be kept below the threshold of 100 mGy, to prevent teratogenic effects on the fetus which can lead to fetal abnormalities, miscarriage, etc.

229:

Answer: D. Patients emotions about pain

Explanation: It is important to assess any type of pain correctly to ensure its proper management. While pain is often subjective, few standard objectives are used to assess it and plan treatment accordingly. WILDA describes an approach where the following factors of pain are assessed- (1) location- where is the pain and if it spreading or localized; (2) intensity- usually measured in adults using a scale 0-10 ; (3) duration- when it occurs, for how long, etc; (4) aggravating and relieving factors- any specific factor/process that causes an increase or decrease in the pain intensity is assessed; (5) words- mainly refers to the description of pain using various words like pricking, throbbing, etc. Proper pain assessment will ensure effective treatment of it. Any feelings of emotions attached to the main are not part of the assessment.

230:
Answer: D.   Its commonly seen in those below 40 years of age
Explanation: Prostate cancer is a common type of cancer seen affecting older men above 50 years of age usually. While there are no symptoms in the early stages, later symptoms present as trouble urinating, blood in urine, decreased force in urine stream, etc. Screening for prostate cancer includes a digital rectal exam (DRE) and Prostate-specific antigen (PSA) test. PSA levels are increased in the blood due to prostate cancer. If screening detects any abnormalities then further diagnostic tools are used like ultrasounds, MRI and biopsy. Low-Grade prostate cancer doesn't require treatment but just constant monitoring, while surgery, radiation therapy, ablative therapies, chemotherapy, hormone therapy, immunotherapy and targeted drug therapy may also be done as needed.

231:
Answer: D.   Antiemetic

Explanation: Ondansetron is a commonly used antiemetic to prevent nausea and vomiting after cancer chemotherapy with agents like cisplatin, surgery or radiation therapy. It is a competitive serotonin type 3 receptor antagonist acting on the central and/or peripheral nervous system. It may be administered as oral tablets, orally disintegrating tablets (ODT), or injections 30-60 mins prior to cancer treatment and then again at regular intervals after the treatment procedure. It is contraindicated in patients taking apomorphine. Side effects that are less severe include headache, constipation, weakness. Severe complications rarely seen include blurred vision, itching, breathing difficulties.

232:
Answer: A.   Goserelin
Explanation: Breast cancer is one of the most common malignancies in women. Those diagnosed at younger ages are positive for hormone receptors and are therefore suitable for endocrine therapy. Upto 90% of the hormones are produced by the ovary and hence ovarian ablation is an important part of endocrine therapy. Luteinizing hormone-releasing hormone agonist therapy, using drugs like goserelin, is recommended in the adjuvant, recurrent, or metastatic settings for premenopausal women with breast cancer.

233:
Answer: D.   Metastatic melanoma
Explanation: Metastatic melanoma is considered to react to treatment with interleukin- This is because metastatic melanoma is known to be sensitive to this type of treatment.

234:
Answer: A.   Are associated with humoral immunity

Explanation: Humoral immunity is mediated by B lymphocytes which are formed and mature in the primary lymphoid tissue, mainly bone marrow. B cells help by producing antibodies and by presenting antigens to various other cells like macrophages, and t-lymphocytes. Thus allowing T-cells to get activated and provide cell-mediated immunity. B-cells differentiate to form various cells like plasma cells, memory B-cells and regulatory B-cells. T- cells may be of two types- helper T-cells or Natural killer cells, both of which help in destroying intracellular pathogens, while B-cells help in the destruction of extracellular pathogens and activation of T-cells also.

235:
Answer: D.   Asbestos
Explanation: Ionizing radiations are a form of energy that is found in both natural (cosmic rays and radon) and manmade (x-rays, radiation therapy, etc) sources. These ionizing radiations can be absorbed by human tissues and cause harmful effects including carcinogenesis. In the United States, radon is the second most common cause of lung cancer. While diagnostic aids like chest x-rays, CT, CBCT, etc expose patients to ionizing radiation. MRI and Ultrasound do not involve ionizing radiations. Asbestos is a type of fibrous mineral found in the soils and rocks which is increasingly linked to cancer.

236:
Answer: D.   Diet
Explanation: Diet plays a significant role in the prevention or causation of colon cancer. Various studies have concluded that a diet rich in vegetables, fruits and whole grains are linked to decreased risk of colon cancer. Decreased consumption of red meat and processed food like white bread is also said to help prevent colon cancer and if consumed in excess can increase the risk for the same. Diet is a modifiable risk factor, whereas age, genetics, race cannot be modified.

237:
Answer: D.   Premature death

Explanation: If someone's end-of-life care is neglected, their premature death is one possible outcome. Other possible outcomes include serious injury or illness, and immense psychological distress. It is important to ensure that all patients receive the necessary end-of-life care in order to ensure their safety and comfort.

238:
Explanation: The nurse's intervention would be to discuss hospice services with William. Hospice services are designed to provide care for patients who are terminally ill and choose to forgo treatment. This type of care can provide significant comfort for the patient and their family in their final days.

239:
Answer: C.   Depression
Explanation: If the nurse is looking for signs of depression in someone, they should look for things like sadness, lack of interest in activities, changes in weight or appetite, difficulty sleeping, and feeling tired all the time.

240:
Answer: D.   Cutting into the center of the tumor
Explanation: Surgical excision of tumors has to be done carefully to prevent the spread of the cancer cells to other sites accidentally. Various steps are undertaken to ensure this and make sure no remnant cancer cells are left behind, which include removal of little normal tissue surrounding the cancer margin , excising cancer tissue from the margins and not cutting across it thus preventing spillage of cancer cells to surrounding tissue, radical surgery involving removal of close by lymph nodes which may be affected, no isolation technique which involves ligation of the primary blood vessels feeding the tumors,and irritation of tumor site with cytotoxic agents.

241:
Answer: C.   50%

Explanation: About half (50%) of cancer deaths can be prevented by adopting a healthy lifestyle and proper access and use of screening for cancer. Lifestyle modifications include avoiding alcohol and tobacco, eating healthy foods, regular physical activity, and proper stress management. Screening is basically testing individuals who have no symptoms of a specific disease. Early detection of cancer through various known screening methods will help reduce deaths due to cancers involving breasts, colon and rectum, lung, etc. Screening also helps in identification and removal of various precancerous lesions.

242:

Answer: C. Meant to provide relief from symptoms and stress of illness

Explanation: Palliative care is offered to patients in various stages of serious illnesses. For cancer patients, it can be offered prior to, during and after treatment also. Palliative care is meant to improve the quality of life of the patient by relieving symptoms and stress of illness. It can be provided in the hospital, at home, at the hospice or in other places too. It is an important duty of the oncology nurse and involves many others including doctors, family and friends, social workers, counselors, alternative medical personnel, spiritual advisor, etc as best suited for the patient. It helps provide relief from physical symptoms like fatigue, nausea, pain, etc, and mental issues like depression, anxiety, and also helps deal with social issues like fear of relations, financial issues.

243:

Answer: B. Not associated with lung cancer or breast cancer

Explanation: Malignant pericardial effusion is a condition in which cancer causes extra fluid to collect in the pericardium and exerts pressure on the heart interfering with its pumping action. Commonly seen in advanced lung cancer, breast cancer, malignant melanoma and leukemia. Symptoms may appear slowly or rapidly, which include dyspnea, chest pain, and cough. Severe cases present with cardiac tamponade and may show tachycardia, decreased heart sounds, peripheral edema, etc, which worsen as the disease progresses. Diagnosis includes chest x-ray showing an enlarged cardiac silhouette and ECG. Treatment includes chemotherapy or radiation therapy for tumors, pericardiocentesis, pericardial sclerosis, Surgical decompression therapies, etc. The treatment chosen depends on tumor and symptom presentation and progression.

244:
Answer: B. Exposure to direct or secondary tobacco smoke.
Explanation: Smoking is the leading cause of lung cancer. Cigarette smoke contains over 7,000 chemicals, including hundreds that are toxic and about 70 that can cause cancer. When you smoke, you inhale all of these chemicals directly into your lungs. Exposure to direct or secondary tobacco smoke is the major cause of lung cancer.

245:
Answer: C. Elderly people
Explanation: Many elderly people are at a higher risk for inadequate pain management due to their age and the health conditions they are often battling. This can lead to increased stress and anxiety levels, and an overall poorer quality of life in their final days.

246:
Answer: C. To arrange a meeting with family members and health care members to discuss patient's wish

Explanation: Robert's son is clearly very involved and passionate about decisions surrounding his father's care. However, it is not appropriate for him to be making all of these decisions unilaterally. The nurse should arrange a meeting with family members and healthcare members to discuss the patient's wishes. This will allow for a more collaborative decision-making process that takes into account all of the relevant parties.

247:
Answer: A.   Impending spinal cord compression

Explanation: The nurse is seeing signs that suggest that William's prostate cancer is progressing and causing compression on his spinal cord. This can lead to pain, bowel dysfunction, and other issues. It is important to monitor William closely and treatment may be necessary to relieve the compression and improve his quality of life.

248:
Answer: C.   Having small meals, scheduled liquids and chewing properly

Explanation: Dumping syndrome is a common complication seen in those who undergo surgery for esophageal cancer. It involves sudden and quick "dumping" of food into the small bowel quickly without being fully digested, which leads to a chemical response that flushes excess water into the intestines. Symptoms include stomach ache, dizziness, diarrhea soon after eating. The exact cause for this is unknown and is said to end with proper recovery and lifestyle adjustments. Managements of this include eating light and small meals, avoiding any triggering food like high-fat food, chewing properly, and scheduling liquids consumption.

249:
Answer: A.   Ovarian cancer

Explanation: There are a few different types of cancer that can be avoided when oral contraceptive pills are used for more than 5 years. The most common type is ovarian cancer. Other types of cancer that can be avoided include uterine cancer and colorectal cancer.

250:
Answer: C.   Exploring the meaning of pain with the patient

Explanation: When a patient refuses to take painkillers because pain is an inevitable part of life, the nurse will likely say something along the lines of exploring the meaning of pain with the patient. This is because the nurse understands that each person experiences pain in different ways and may find relief in different ways. By exploring the meaning of pain with the patient, the nurse can help identify any underlying issues that may be causing them to feel resistant to taking painkillers.

251:
Answer: A.   Antihistamines

Explanation: If a cancer patient develops itching (pruritus), one possible treatment is to give them an antihistamine. Antihistamines are drugs that block the action of histamine, which is a chemical that can cause itching.

252:
Answer: B. Osteoporosis

Explanation: Aromatase inhibitors are used to treat breast cancer and they are potent estrogen inhibitors. There are two types - nonsteroidal reversible inhibitors and steroidal irreversible inhibitors. Estrogen has antiresorptive effects on osteoclasts during bone remodeling and aromatase inhibitors prevent this action causing bone loss and osteoporosis. As antiresorptive agents, oral and iv bisphosphonates can be given along with aromatase inhibitors.

253:
Answer: A.   ABVD

Explanation: Hodgkin's lymphoma is treated using various combinations of chemotherapy and/or radiation therapy. Treatment of HL is known to affect male fertility i.e. spermatogenesis to various degrees. ABVD is combination chemotherapy that uses Adriamycin, bleomycin, vinblastine, dacarbazine and is proven to have the least detrimental effect on fertility. Side effects to spermatogenesis are seen max at six months post-treatment and recovery is seen 12-24 months post-treatment, also with an improvement in those who had pretreatment impaired spermatogenesis. Other combination chemotherapies like MOPP, BEACOPP, etc have reportedly caused worse effects on male fertility with low and late recovery rates.

254:
Answer: A. Encouraging a high-fat diet and bed rest
Explanation: Bowel obstruction may be complete or partial, Mechanical or functional and affects the small bowel 90% of the time. Nursing management includes various processes like:
- encouraging the patient to have a high fiber diet and exercise regularly which help in the movement of contents through the bowel properly
- continuous assessment of pain and progress of the patient through bowel auscultation and palpation;
- looking for dehydration signs like chapped lips, swollen tongue, etc
- keeping patient on Fowler's or semi-fowlers position (45-60 degrees) to ease respiratory distress due to distended abdomen
- insert NG tube if needed; monitor patient fluid and electrolyte balance
- provide post-op care as needed
- assess for signs of peritonitis like fever, abdominal rigidity

255:
Answer: C. The nurse can ask his parents to leave a message as they are not allowed to meet him
Explanation: If a gay man is near death due to leukemia and his parents will not accept his lifestyle or lover, he can ask the hospice not to allow them to visit him in his room. The nurse's best course of action is to respect the patient's wishes and ask his parents to leave a message.

256:
Answer: D. Increased energy

Explanation: Depression is a serious psychological illness that affects life negatively. It varies from mild to severe depression. People have feelings of sadness, hopelessness, guilt, lack of interest in anything, lack of energy to do routine things or activities previously interested in, loss of appetite and weight loss, and insomnia. Suicidal thoughts may also be experienced by some. These feelings are not for merely a day but are continuous for over two weeks in depressed people. Treatment includes pharmacological drugs like antidepressants, alternative therapies like music therapy, counseling, etc. It's important to clearly note the patient's history in such cases to know about previous similar episodes and/or treatments being used for the same. Various factors that affect depression in an individual include genetics, violent environment, and low self-esteem.

257:
Answer: B. Condom used during sexual activities

Explanation: Those who have AIDS are at a higher risk for several AIDS-defining malignancies including Kaposi sarcoma, non-Hodgkin lymphoma [NHL], invasive cervical cancer, and also non-AIDS-defining malignancies (NADMs). 33 percent of HIV-positive deaths are due to cancer. While antiretroviral therapy (ART) Is needed to treat HIV, chemotherapy is required to treat cancer. Avoiding sexual activities while ideal may not be a practical choice. Unprotected sex is strictly prohibited because of the risk of the spread of AIDS and/or chemotherapy agents also. The use of a condom during sexual intercourse or oral sex also helps to reduce the risk of infection. While ART may lower the viral load and make the person not infective, it is still advised to use a condom.

258:
Answer: D. Mood swings, increased hunger, double vision

Explanation: Insulinoma is a tumor of the pancreas which secretes increased amounts of insulin. This increased insulin level leads to hypoglycemia (decreased blood sugar) and its associated symptoms including confusion, sweating, weakness, rapid heartbeat, double vision, mood swings, hunger etc. Treatment usually involves surgical removal of the tumor. Management involves medication, frequent meals, etc.

259:
Answer: D.   Axillary node dissection
Explanation: The chance of developing lymphedema after breast cancer surgery increases significantly when the axillary node dissection is performed. This is because the removal of lymph nodes in the armpit can damage the network of lymphatic vessels and ducts that help drain fluid from the arm and hand. As a result, excess fluid may accumulate and cause swelling in the arm and hand.

260:
Answer: D. Cisplatin
Explanation: Nitrogen mustard is an antineoplastic, alkylating drug. Nitrogen mustard agents act by alkylating DNA of the cancer cells thus slowing down or stopping cancer cells' growth and replication because of DNA strand breakage of cross-linking of 2 strands. Mechlorethamine, Cyclophosphamide, Chlorambucil, Melphalan, and Ifosfamide are all mustard gas derivatives. Cisplatin is a metal salt. Nitrogen mustard is normally administered IV or its lotion is applied on the skin to treat mycosis fungoides skin lesions. Side effects may occur like low blood count, nausea, hair loss, darkening of veins used for IV administration, etc. It is used as a combination treatment for various cancers, as palliative care, or as a lotion for mycosis fungoides skin lesions.

261:
Answer: D.   Both radioactive or chemotherapy agents can be added to it to cause targeted cell destruction

Explanation: Monoclonal antibodies are of various types that are- naked monoclonal antibodies and conjugated monoclonal antibodies. Conjugated monoclonal antibodies aka labeled or tagged antibodies are basically a type of monoclonal antibody which bind to various cell surface antigens but are not toxic to the cell, unlike unconjugated/naked monoclonal antibodies. CMA is combined with either a chemotherapy drug or radioactive particles which are delivered to specific cells directly thus causing the least damage to normal cells. Ibritumomab tiuxetan is a conjugated mAb that has both a drug and a radioactive substance attached to it. Examples of chemo-labeled conjugated mAb include brentuximab and TDM.

262:
Answer: B. Talk to the patient about these feelings and fears, suggest basic coping mechanisms, and evaluate the patient
Explanation: Coping basically refers to changing cognitive and behavioral efforts to maintain change in internal and/or external demands. Cancer patients face huge changes in their personal and professional lives with the diagnosis and treatment. Emotional, mental, physical, and spiritual aspects of their lives undergo changes and it's important the patient learns to cope with these changes in a healthy manner. Feelings like frustration, anxiety, worry, etc are common and nurses must discuss such emotions with the patient freely instead of avoiding such topics. Nurses must regularly evaluate the patient's coping through observation, conversations, and questionnaires like COPE, or WCQ. Only if needed must the physician or psychiatrist be asked to intervene with medication or counseling. Encouraging the patient to cope with the cancer diagnosis and treatment initially includes talking to their family, family, spiritual practices, and alternative therapies.

263:
Answer: A. Hypertonic saline via continuous infusion

Explanation: Low sodium levels in patients with small cell lung cancer can occur due to various reasons, out of which syndrome of inadequate antidiuretic hormone secretion (SIADH) is the most common. While it may be asymptomatic, symptoms like nausea, fatigue, headache, seizures, cramps, etc may be seen in the patient. The first line of emergency treatment in such cases is the administration of hypertonic saline via a continuous solution which will improve the patient's general condition and neurological state. Drugs that may be used for the treatment of this later include demeclocycline which negates the effect of ADH but its effects are delayed for 1-2 weeks and vasopressin receptor antagonists like conivaptan,and tolvaptan.

264:
Answer: A.   Loperamide
Explanation: Loperamide is a medication that is used to treat radiation-induced diarrhea. It helps to control diarrhea by slowing down the smooth muscle movement in the intestines. This helps to reduce the number of bowel movements and helps to make them less watery.

265:
Answer: B.   No change in fertility
Explanation: The nurse's reaction will be no change in fertility. When a man has testicular cancer, one of the treatments can be a unilateral orchiectomy, which is the removal of one testicle. This surgery will not affect the man's fertility.

266:
Answer: D. Not talking about her grief and being normal

Explanation: Grief is a normal emotional response and it is important that the person grieving goes through a healthy process of grief. Normal grief responses which include sadness, guilt, and missing feelings must be dealt with in a healthy manner. There is no specific timeline but prolonged and extreme grief even after 6-12 months may require special attention and interventions. Grief can be dealt with properly by expressing feelings and thoughts to family and friends, following specific religious and spiritual customs that the person believes in, counseling with a professional, and support groups. Denying feelings and substance abuse with alcohol or drugs and self-harm are strictly prohibited as they do not help the person through their grieving process but only worsen the condition and help them avoid the situation instead of deal with it.

267:
Answer: B.   Administering dexrazoxane
Explanation: Dexrazoxane is a cardiac protective agent that is often given to patients who are receiving doxorubicin. This agent helps to protect the heart from the toxic effects of doxorubicin.

268:
Answer: C. Originally derived from Streptomyces peucetius
Explanation: Doxorubicin is an anthracycline antibiotic originally derived from Streptomyces peucetius and it has antineoplastic activity. It acts by intercalation with DNA thus preventing protein synthesis, inhibiting the enzyme Topoisomerase II and forming oxygen-free radicals. The oxygen-free radicals formed may lead to oxidative stress which contributes to the most dangerous side effect of the drug which is dilated cardiomyopathy. Other side effects include red color urine, inflammation of the bowel, PPE, alopecia. Doxorubicin is administered intravenously. Various cancers treated using this drug include kaposi's sarcoma, breast cancer, and bladder cancer.

269:
Answer: C. Both are reversible

Explanation: Many advanced cancer patients undergo a wasting syndrome characterized by anorexia and cachexia. While anorexia refers to loss of appetite and/or aversion to food and cachexia refers to the loss of body mass. Both are often associated with weakness, fatigue, poor quality of life etc. Both of these can be managed and usually reversed with adequate care. Management involves nutritional counseling where small multiple meals are advised, avoiding spicy foods, and also use of appetite stimulants like corticosteroids and progestational agents such as megestrol and medroxyprogesterone can lead to appetite stimulation and weight gain. Enteral and parenteral nutrition is also advised. Psychological counseling may also be required for the patient. Family and friends must also be advised on how to handle such situations.

270:
Answer: A.   Control in cancer growth
Explanation: The goal of treatment with fluorouracil and leucovorin is to control the growth of the tumor.

271:
Answer: C. Given as subcutaneous/iv injections 24 hours after chemotherapy
Explanation: Cancer patients may be given granulocyte colony-stimulating factor (G-CSF) (generic name- filgrastim; trade name-Neupogen) to reduce the incidence of infection or fever, collect WBC prior to bone marrow transplantation and to improve high-dose radiation outcome. It basically stimulates the growth of neutrophils, a type of WBC. It is administered as an injection under the skin or into the vein. Side effects of this include bone pain, low platelet count, allergic reactions, dizziness, fever, pain at the injection site, symptoms of kidney injury like red/brown urine, etc. Conceiving a child is NOT allowed while using this and breastfeeding requires doctors' consultation.

272:
Answer: C.   Cytarabine

Explanation: Cytarabine is a chemotherapy medicine used to treat lymphoma meningitis. It is a type of chemotherapy called an antimetabolite, which means it interferes with the growth of cancer cells.

273:
Answer: A. African-Americans are at a greater risk for it than other races
Explanation: Colon cancer is said to usually affect older men. Risk factors for colon cancer include low fiber and high fat diets, African-American race, colon polyps, family history, and inflammatory bowel diseases. Symptoms of colon cancer include alterations in bowel movements including diarrhea or constipation and change in stool consistency, blood in stools, rectal bleeding, abdominal discomfort, sudden weight loss, and weakness. In the earlier stages of the disease, few or no symptoms may be experienced. Staging will help determine the treatment plan and it ranges from 0-IV. By stage IV, metastasis of the cancer is seen.

274:
Answer: D.   Renal disease
Explanation: The patient's symptoms may be indicative of malignant ascites, which is a complication of certain cancers, including lung cancer. One measure that can be taken to reduce the risk of developing malignant ascites is to treat any underlying renal disease. This can help to improve the function of the kidneys and reduce the amount of tumor-related waste products that build up in the body.

275:

Answer: B. tumor lysis syndrome
Explanation: When cancer cells break down quickly during chemotherapy, there is a rise in uric acid, phosphorus and potassium levels in the body, which affect various organs such as kidneys, heart, and brain. Symptoms experienced are usually nonspecific and include nausea, lack of appetite, dark urine, reduced urine output, hallucinations, and muscle cramps. Treatment and prevention include iv fluids, allopurinol. Blood tests are done regularly to assess electrolyte levels and damage to various organs.

276:
Answer: A. About half an hour after a meal
Explanation: When a person is on pain medications, their bowel function can be affected. This can lead to constipation and stool retention. In order to help William start bowel evacuation, you should help him sit on a toilet or commode about half an hour after he has eaten.

277:
Answer: B.   Chronic Myeloid leukemia
Explanation: Chronic myeloid leukemia (CML) is a type of cancer that starts in the blood-forming cells of the bone marrow. In CML, a type of white blood cell called a myeloid cell becomes abnormal and grows out of control. These abnormal cells can spread to other parts of the body such as the lymph nodes, spleen, liver, and brain. CML is treated with allogeneic stem cell transplantation, which is a treatment that replaces unhealthy blood-forming cells with healthy ones from a donor.

278:
Answer: D. level of health literacy
Explanation: Health literacy refers to an individual's ability to access, understand, appraise, and apply health-related information. According to various studies, health literacy is said to greatly influence cancer patients' behavior and how they use the health services available. Inadequate health literacy is associated with unfavorable health outcomes. Hence it is important that oncology nurses be aware of the patient's health literacy to assess their adherence to treatment plans and if needed educate the patients about health, and need for treatment which will remove any barriers to patient's treatment and recovery.

279:
Answer: C. Dosage is administered as prescribed

Explanation: Various studies have shown that food affects the bioavailability of chlorambucil. The peak plasma levels and elimination rate of chlorambucil were reduced when taken along with food, which affects the drug action and dosage needed. Hence it is advised to take chlorambucil on an empty stomach, with 1 hour before a meal or 2 hours after meals. The medication must be swallowed as a whole orally and not be crushed, chewed, or broken.

280:
Answer: C. Erythema multiforme
Explanation: Erythema multiforme is a hypersensitive reaction leading to characteristic target skin lesions that may have various triggers which include certain drugs, viral infections, cancer, etc. It is usually self limiting once the causative factor has been removed. The combination of chemotherapy and radiation has been known to cause EM. Lesions usually begin to appear over irradiated areas of the skin and then spread. Reduced immunity during cancer and its treatment also leads to a number of viral and bacterial infections which can trigger EM. While it usually resolves on its own, steroids, pain medication and bandaging may be required for the lesions.

281:
Answer: A. organ metastasis
Explanation: Metastasis of cancer is when cancer cells break off from the initial tumor site and travel through the blood or lymph and form new tumors in different sites. This metastasis of cancer cells into other organs and the blood disrupts organ functions and destroys the healthy cells, oxygen supply, blood supply. The occurrence of this in vital organs may be the most common cause of death in patients with cancer.

282:
Answer: D.   High dose chemotherapy

Explanation: A myeloablation procedure is a medical treatment that destroys the patient's bone marrow. The goal of a myeloablation procedure is to remove the patient's bone marrow before they undergo a stem cell transplant. This eliminates any cancerous cells that may be present in the bone marrow and helps to improve the chances that the stem cell transplant will be successful.

283:
Answer: A. Lung cancer
Explanation: Pruritus is an itchy feeling on the skin that makes a person scratch their skin and may also feel pain. Generalized pruritus may be the first sign of cancer in some cases and is also a side effect of cancer treatment. Leukemia, lymphoma, and liver cancer are the most common cancers associated with itching. It is said to occur due to the direct presence of cancer in the skin or metastasis to skin, which may lead to build up of bile salts or maybe due to substances secreted by the tumor or the body in response to the tumor. Chemotherapy-related itching may suggest sensitivity to the drug being used and radiation therapy may kill cancer cells causing drying, itching and burning of the skin. High doses of these treatments are more commonly associated with pruritus. Certain drugs used in immunotherapy may also cause pruritus. While pruritus may be seen with other cancers also, lung cancer is not commonly associated with this symptom.

284:
Answer: A. Creatinine clearance
Explanation: Zoledronic is a bisphosphonate that helps lower blood calcium levels. Various studies have proven a major side effect of the drug is renal toxicity, the chances of which are more in patients with pre-existing medical conditions, old age. To reduce the risk of adverse renal effects, it is advised to check the creatinine clearance of the patient to assess renal function. If the value is less than 35mL/min then zoledronic acid is not administered to the patient.

285:
Answer: B. Bone marrow transplant

Explanation: Cancer treatment in both males and females may affect their sexuality also. Various procedures that involve sexual organs like the vagina, vulva, etc and also other surgeries like mastectomy that affect the appearance of the individual affect the sexual activity of the patient. Radical cystectomy involves the removal of the bladder, uterus, ovaries, fallopian tubes, cervix, front wall of the vagina, and the urethra. Bilateral oophorectomy involves the removal of both the ovaries. Mastectomy involves the removal of the entire breast. Bone marrow transplant surgery is a procedure that infuses healthy blood-forming stem cells into the patient's body to replace the diseased bone marrow, thus having the least effect on the sexuality of the patient.

286:
Answer: D. Radical cystectomy
Explanation: Noninvasive bladder cancer is when cancer cells are found only in the inner lining of the bladder. Transurethral resection of bladder tumor (TURBT) is a common surgical method done which makes use of a cystoscope inserted into the urethra and the bladder, and the tumor is removed or fulguration may also be done. Bacillus Calmette-Guérin (BCG) is a vaccine that helps stop or delay bladder cancer and hence can be given once a week for 6 weeks after TURT as a treatment modality. Intravesical chemotherapy is where a chemotherapeutic drug is directly placed into the patient's bladder using a catheter. Radical cystectomy is the removal of the whole bladder and also nearby lymph nodes which is done only for invasive bladder cancer.

287:
Answer: C. lung cancer

Explanation: Prophylactic surgery for cancer involves surgery done to prevent cancer in certain organs of the body in individuals who are at high risk of that specific cancer. Prophylactic mastectomy is a common procedure done where the breast tissue is removed to prevent breast cancer. It is commonly done in individuals with mutations in BRCA1 and BRCA2 genes, a history of cancer in one breast, etc. Prophylactic salpingectomy involves the removal of fallopian tubes and prophylactic oophorectomy involves the removal of ovaries, both procedures help reduce the risk of ovarian cancer. Prophylactic colectomy involves the removal of part of the colon to prevent colon cancer. Prophylactic surgery of vital organs like lungs, liver, etc is not yet done.

288:
Answer: B. II
Explanation: Clinical trials are basically designed to ensure that new treatments are better than existing therapies for various diseases. Various phases of the clinical trial are as follows- 1) phase I - the safety of a drug, appropriate dosage and route of administration is determined and it includes a smaller number of people; 2) phase 2 - usually includes less than 100 people and is meant to test if the drug works for a specific disease; 3) phase III - tests if the new treatment is better than standard treatment; 4) phase 4 - here FDA approved treatments are continued to be studied for long term side effects

289:
Answer: D. Analysing success/failure rates for various treatment options
Explanation: Cancer survivors need to take care even after the completion of successful treatment. They often need additional support easing back into their regular life. Oncology nurses are meant to help them through the process and follow up on their health status. During the assessment of the oncology survivor, nurses must get to know about the patient's disease, treatment type and its effects, support systems, available resources for the management of side effects, mental health of patient, etc. Excessive critiquing of the reason for a patient choosing a specific treatment and its statistics must not be discussed with the patient as it may hurt, anger or annoy the patient and create a lack of understanding between the nurse and the patient.

290:
Answer: D.   **The physician has explained all these to my family**

Explanation: A clinical trial participant has made an informed decision when he understands the risks and benefits of the clinical trial and what is involved in being a participant. The best description of this would be when the participant's physician has explained everything to their family and they are fully aware of what taking part in the trial would entail.

291:
Answer: B: Avoid thiazide diuretics

Explanation: Thiazides may commonly cause an increase in blood calcium levels due to promoting the reabsorption of calcium in distal tubules to reduce urinary calcium. For those at risk of hypercalcemia, this can be highly dangerous and hence they must avoid the consumption of thiazide diuretics. Thiazide-associated hypercalcemia has been seen more commonly in women than men and its incidence increases with age.

292:
Answer: B. Effects of tumor and treatment causes issues like GI troubles, etc which cause sleep disturbances

Explanation: Sleep disorders are very common in cancer patients. It may be due to the cancer diagnosis, the tumor or treatment. Cancer diagnosis may cause stress and anxiety in the patient and result in insomnia. Tumors may have various effects which include GI disturbances, pain, fever, itching, or bladder problems which will in turn cause sleep issues. Treatments may also lead to various side effects like pain, bladder issues, or fever which cause sleep disturbances. Certain medications used commonly affect cancer treatment like corticosteroids, hormone therapy, and antidepressants. Hospital environments also make it difficult to sleep properly due to constant disturbances by doctors and nurses, new surroundings, or uncomfortable beds.

293:
Answer: D. use of alcohol

Explanation: Anxiety and distress are commonly seen in cancer survivors. Fears in those treated for cancer include fear of cancer recurrence, concerns about family, finances, body image, and sexuality. It is important that the patient finds ways and learns to cope with such fears in a healthy manner. Various methods include cognitive behavioral therapy, exercise, support groups, mindfulness-based stress reduction, and self-management. Use of alcohol or drugs is strictly prohibited. Medications are also supposed to be used only according to the doctor's prescription, instead of abused as a coping mechanism.

294:
Answer: B. Educate the patient about body image and provide encouraging words
Explanation: Body image difficulties are commonly seen in cancer patients who undergo various treatments and are most prevalent immediately postoperatively and during the treatment. Neck dissection and mandibulectomy will lead to significant changes in the patient's appearance, and hence the psychosocial aspect of it will include body image issues. Nurses can best help promote a positive body image in such patients by offering words of support and encouragement, educating the patient about these aspects of treatment, providing patients with the information they need to deal with the changes, and treating them normally. This includes being present with the patient when he first looks in the mirror post-treatment and guiding them through the process of having a positive body image.

295:

Answer: D. CT

Explanation: Increased intracranial pressure is a neurological emergency in cancer patients. There are many reasons for increased ICP in cancer patients like brain tumors exerting pressure on the skull, tumor causing vasogenic edema, robust inflammatory reaction 3-6 months after radiotherapy, etc. There are various imaging techniques to assess the brain tumor like CT, MRI, DSA and various other advances like CT angiography, diffusion weighted imaging (DWI), functional MRI, etc. CT is considered the most rapid imaging technique which shows internal body structures like tissues, organs and skeletal structures. It is faster and cheaper compared to MRI but MRI helps in more detailed imaging.

296:

Answer: A.   Methotrexate
Explanation: Various drugs are given to a cancer patient during chemotherapy that is meant to target the cancer cells but unfortunately they do have few negative effects on other cells. The liver is one such organ in the body that may get adversely affected due to long term use of certain medications in cancer patients. Out of the mentioned drugs, methotrexate is the drug most likely to lead to fatty liver, liver fibrosis, and cirrhosis on long term use. It is known to cause serum aminotransferase elevations. With long term, low-to-moderate dose methotrexate therapy, elevations in serum ALT or AST is seen in about 15% to 50% of the patients which is usually of low-to-moderate risk. Hence those on long term chemotherapy are advised to get regular follow-ups to assess any side effects that may appear due to treatment.

297:
Answer: B.   Axillary node dissection
Explanation: The chance of developing lymphedema after breast cancer surgery increases significantly when the axillary node dissection is performed. This is because the removal of lymph nodes in the armpit can damage the network of lymphatic vessels and ducts that help drain fluid from the arm and hand. As a result, excess fluid may accumulate and cause swelling in the arm and hand.

298:

Answer: A. Oral phosphodiesterase type 5 inhibitors

Explanation: Erectile dysfunction is common in cancer patients, as chemotherapy and radiation therapy can damage the nerves and blood vessels necessary for an erection. Oral phosphodiesterase type 5 inhibitors, such as sildenafil (Viagra), tadalafil (Cialis), and vardenafil (Levitra), are the most effective treatment for erectile dysfunction and have the best chance of helping the patient. These medications work by blocking the enzyme that breaks down cGMP, the molecule responsible for smooth muscle relaxation and erection.

Dear Nurse,

Thank you for taking the time to read this book.

We know you could have chosen any number of books to read, but you picked this one, and we are very grateful.

We hope that you found this book to be a helpful resource in your OCN Exam preparation. If you are happy with it and found it beneficial in some way, we'd like to hear from you. Please take a moment to post a review on Amazon. Your feedback and support will help us to make this book even better and improve our writing for future projects.

Your review is very important to us as it helps us morally and persuades us to do better each time. Hope this book helped you in some way to crack the OCN exam.

All the best for your exam. Do it with confidence. Think and recall what you have learned and then answer the questions. You will surely be a proud and caring OCN.

Warm Regards,
Prof. Winifred Taylor
& Pro Oncologist Team

Made in the USA
Coppell, TX
06 August 2022